Chicken Soup for the Soul
Healthy Living:
Breast Cancer

Chicken Soup for the Soul
Healthy Living:
Breast Cancer

Jack Canfield

Mark Victor Hansen

Mary Olsen Kelly

Edward Creagan, M.D.
CANCER SPECIALIST, MAYO CLINIC

Health Communications, Inc.
Deerfield Beach, Florida

www.bcibooks.com
www.chickensoup.com

We would like to acknowledge the many publishers and individuals who granted us permission to reprint the cited material.

The Best Thing That Ever Happened to Me. Reprinted by permission of Vicki Rackner, M.D. © 2004 Vicki Rackner.

No Mountain Too High. Reprinted by permission of Michele V. Price. © 2004 Michele V. Price.

Leave 'em Laughing. Reprinted by permission of Lillie Shockney. © 2000 Lillie Shockney. Originally published in *Voices from the Edge.* Michael H. Samuelson.

Barney. Reprinted by permission of Mary Ellen LaFavers. © 2003 Mary Ellen LaFavers.

(Continues on page 130)

Library of Congress Cataloging-in-Publication Data
available from the Library of Congress

Publisher: Health Communications, Inc.
3201 S.W. 15th Street
Deerfield Beach, FL 33442-8190

Cover design by Larissa Hise Henoch
Inside book design by Lawna Patterson Oldfield

Contents

Fear less, hope more,

eat less, chew more,

whine less, breathe more,

talk less, say more,

love more,

and all good things

will be yours.

—Swedish Proverb

Introduction:

You Can Survive Any Diagnosis

"*My world turned upside down at seven o'clock on the morning of March 8 as I stood in the shower.*" A lump in the breast. A moment of panic. So begins a journey that every woman fears.

We all know the statistics; we all know the numbers. More women die of heart disease than breast cancer. But no disease strikes a dagger into the soul of a woman like breast cancer.

"*I finally mustered the courage to call my husband at work. He was stunned. Neither of us knew what to do. As the day wore on, I again felt my breast and realized my worst fears. Yes, the mass was still there. Like most of us, I rationalized, I bargained, I willed it to go away: This must be due to my period. It must be a cyst. It must be an injury while cleaning the house.*

"*I called my doctor who agreed to see me several days down the road. Obviously, this was unacceptable. I told his office staff that I was on my way over, and I would sit in his office until he examined me and decided what to do. Thus began one of the most painful, challenging, and yet liberating, experiences of my life.*"

Liberating, you ask?

How can getting a life-threatening disease such as breast cancer be liberating?

I have seen this liberating power in my clinical practice. My breast cancer patients view life with new lenses. Time takes on new meaning. What's important in life takes center stage—even if that means changing jobs, dumping a husband, marrying the long-time boyfriend, moving up a wedding date or launching children who have been hanging around the house too long.

Breast cancer brings insight into the real meaning and purpose of life. Breast cancer opens chapters for each of us as we take the journey—each in our different ways. I learn from my patients about optimism, hope, dedication and love every day.

Patients ask me why. "Why did I get breast cancer?" Rather than waste precious moments wondering whether your illness was caused by something you did or didn't do, or worrying that your mother, sister or daughter will develop breast cancer if yours is a new case in the family, spend your time wisely looking forward and moving on. Only 5 to 10 percent of breast cancer has a genetic origin. For the rest, don't ask why, because there simply is no "why."

The stories we have collected here will inspire you. You'll cry, you'll laugh, but above all, you will feel empowered to make responsible and thoughtful decisions for the most important race of your life and the lives of women you love.

The race for health and wellness is winnable, and it is achievable, but none of us can do it alone. Without friends and family and companions and, above all, information, we are wandering in the medical and spiritual wilderness. In your treatment journey and to sustain you each wonderful day after diagnosis, you will want to use some of the tools we present, including social support, humor, chanting, visual imagery and even the magical healing power of your pet.

The bottom line is simple: health is our most precious gift. To preserve it, as patients, we need to be active, we need to be assertive, and we need to partner with our health care providers and our loved ones. The information in this book may well save your life, may indeed increase the quality of your life and is certainly the best investment you will ever make. I promise.

Edward T. Creagan, M.D.
American Cancer Society Professor of Clinical Oncology
John and Roma Rouse Professor of Humanism in Medicine
Professor, Mayo Clinic College of Medicine

☥

The Best Thing That Ever Happened to Me

My cancer scare changed my life.
I'm grateful for every new, healthy day I have.
It has helped me prioritize my life.

—OLIVIA NEWTON-JOHN, SINGER

I t was late afternoon. I was catching up with my dictation after a busy day of operating, seeing my hospitalized postoperative patients, and evaluating the young and old in my clinic. I am a surgeon, and my mission, as taught in medical school and surgical residency, is to cure by cutting out disease.

Maxine, my office manager, poked her head in the door. "Claire just got through seeing her oncologist and stopped in to say hi. Is this a good time?" Claire and I have a deep connection. I have accompanied her on an arduous journey with painful twists and turns.

About two years earlier, Claire found out her husband was having an affair. She took herself to a nice resort to get away and gain some perspective. As she was soaking in the candlelit tub, she found a lump in her left breast. She said it was as if someone had directed her hand to that spot. She had an ominous feeling, so she cut her trip short.

The day I first met Claire, I examined her breasts. The surgery textbooks describe the feel of cancer: gritty and hard with an irregular, rough surface. *Cancer* is Latin for *crab,* and breast cancer sends out crablike tentacles. The books don't instruct you to listen to your intuition as you do the examination, so I learned to do that on my own. We physicians don't usually offer treatment based on "hunches," so I put a needle in her breast and aspirated cells for the pathologists to look at under the microscope. As I had suspected, there were cancer cells.

How do you tell someone she has breast cancer? There's no easy way, and each doctor finds one that seems best. When I performed Claire's biopsy, I asked her whether she wanted to hear the results over the phone or in person. The next day I called and said, "Claire, this is the phone call you don't want to get." Delivering bad news is the hardest part of being a surgeon. It's easier with a breast cancer patient like Claire because she often knows long before the biopsy results arrive.

Now, two years later and with a cancer-free bill of health from her oncologist, Claire started her victory dance in my office and sang, "Yup. I'm calling some girlfriends, and we're going out on the town." After a moment of reflection, and with all sincerity, out came these words: "Getting breast cancer is the best thing that ever happened to me."

I was not surprised to hear Claire say this. She is the eternal optimist, finding the silver lining with the determination and skill of Sherlock Holmes. Leave it to Claire to frame her story of personal betrayal, disfiguring operations, and chemotherapy and radiation as an opportunity for growth.

"The moment I found my lump in the bathtub, I knew it was cancer. I thought breast cancer was a death sentence," she confided in me. "I didn't know that most women who get breast cancer live a long life. But you know, the woman I was two years ago died. And then the real me was born."

Claire made big changes after her diagnosis. She divorced her husband and dyed her new post-chemotherapy hair blond. She understood both in her head and in her heart that the only moment she is promised is the one she's living. She was going to make each moment count.

♥ *Vicki Rackner, M.D.*

✗ *Think about* . . .
what breast cancer means to me

- ✗ How do I schedule my life around treatment?

- ✗ How do I tell my kids? Will they understand?

- ✗ Will my husband still find me attractive?

- ✗ What do I tell my employer? Should I continue working through treatment? What options do I have?

- ✗ How can I be sure my doctor is offering me the best treatment for my type of breast cancer? Should I get a second opinion now?

- ✗ After surgery, what will I look like? How will I manage the pain?

- ✗ What clothes will I be able to wear?

- ✗ Will I lose my hair?

We all have fears and questions. You can't always control the ones above (but as we'll show, you often can); you *can* always control the answers to the two most important questions you'll ever ask yourself:

- ✗ What does this cancer journey mean to me?

- ✗ How can I make breast cancer "the best thing that ever happened to me"?

The Real Numbers

Even though breast cancer is expected to account for nearly 32 percent of all new cancer cases among women, and just over 668,000 women are diagnosed with some form of cancer each year, long-term survival rates for breast cancer are continuing an upward trend. Some 88 percent of white women and 74 percent of African American women will be able to say that they are "former breast cancer patients."

Lung cancer, not breast cancer, is the leading cause of cancer death among women. Heart disease, not breast cancer, is the leading cause of death among women.

ξ

No Mountain Too High

Cancer wakes you up, and you say,
"There must be more out there to life.
I wonder what that is."

—JILL EIKENBERRY, ACTRESS

W*hat am I doing here?* I ask myself as I stand on the edge of the cliff, close my eyes, position my feet on the edge and lean back into empty space. I take the first step backward over the edge, the ropes at once moving and supporting me. Talking to myself alleviates my fear, and I silently recite the instructions: *Feet flat on rocks; pretend shoes have suction cups; allow rope to slide through hands; feet shoulder-width apart; don't forget, right hand pulled to hip is the brake.* I'm terrified and don't know if I can take another step.

▄▄▄

Just weeks out of chemotherapy for breast cancer recurrence, I stand in the lobby of the hotel, waiting for the van that will transport our cancer survivor group high into the Rockies. The recurrence has left me shaken, and I need to throw myself back into life and regain my courage.

Bus after bus arrives, loads and departs, and my anxiety increases as the lobby empties. Only a few people remain. We stare at one another for a moment and then converge on the center of the room. A young man about thirty looks at me questioningly and asks, "Cancer group?"

"Yes," I reply, relieved to know I'm not alone.

"Emilio," he says and extends his hand. The others follow his lead, and we eagerly shake hands and exchange names.

At last the van arrives, and we begin the two-hour trip to the expedition's center, high in the Colorado mountains. Excitement, apprehension, fear and hope emanate from these strangers, who reflect my own emotions. To succeed on this three-day adventure, we must learn to trust one another very quickly. Cancer is the only thing we presently have in common.

***

I'm balanced on the highest of several narrow steps that are nailed to a tree. Below, my companions stand in two rows, forming a human net with their arms. *Whoever thought of this exercise?* I ask myself as my body hugs the tree. *I've just met these people—can I depend on them to keep my still-fragile body from hitting the ground?*

They speak encouraging words, "Don't think about it; just let go. You didn't drop anyone when you were part of the net."

I close my eyes and breathe deeply—ten breaths, fifteen breaths. I lean back, free-falling safely into the human net.

The fear I experienced during the free fall returns as I lean over the cliff. *Breathe*, I tell myself. My body relaxes, as do my lungs, and once again I lean out and back, allowing the rope to move me slowly downward. Just as I'm gaining confidence, I place my feet too close together, and I swing to one side, almost losing control. I bring my feet to the rocks, stabilizing my swinging body. Though shaken, I feel an unexpected surge of excitement and energy. My feet make friends with the rocks; my body melts into the rope; I experience unencumbered freedom, rappelling for sixty feet.

After a solo night in the woods, loaded with back-packs and sleeping bags, we begin the descent down the steep mountain trail. We don't want this time to end and reluctantly follow the path through the trees, across a wooden bridge and along the creek. Unexpectedly, John turns off the path and leads us to a solid wooden structure nearly twenty feet high.

"This is the wall," he says solemnly. "You have

forty-five minutes to get everyone, leaders included, up and over. No ropes or belts allowed, and no using the sides of the wall." He instructs us to put on our harnesses then calmly walks away to talk with the other counselors. We are left to wonder whether anyone has ever really completed this exercise.

After a few false starts, we begin to focus on the task. Emilio and Tara serve as ladders as we hoist Diane onto their shoulders.

Extending as high as she can on her toes, Diane finally grasps the top board and pulls herself up and over the wall onto the narrow platform behind it. I'm next to climb the human ladder. Diane leans over the wall from the platform and grabs my extended wrists. I dangle in space as I attempt to swing my leg to the edge. At last, I swing high enough for Diane to release one of my hands, grab my leg and haul me over the top. One by one, my companions traverse the wall, until only John and Emilio remain.

Emilio climbs on John's shoulders and reaches for Tara and Diane's extended hands. They grasp his hands, and Emilio dangles as John jumps and grabs his harness, unsuccessfully trying several times to climb up and over him. John continues to slip, and we aren't certain he'll make it. We cheer him on, and gaining renewed energy, he at last pulls himself up and over Emilio, making it to the top.

Together, we hoist the hanging, stretched Emilio to the platform, finishing our task with five minutes to spare, and with the invaluable knowledge that the only walls in life are those we construct ourselves—that cancer doesn't define who we are or determine what we can accomplish.

♥ *Michele V. Price*

Nine Essential Steps to Thriving with Breast Cancer

1. KNOW YOUR DIAGNOSIS

If you can see the enemy, you can fight it. So insist on seeing your X-rays, lab results, CT scans, mammograms, bone scans and MRIs. Acknowledge the seriousness of your diagnosis. This involves knowing the name of the cancer under the microscope, the size and grade of the tumor, and whether this is viewed as slow growing or as an angry process.

Bring in a family member or friend who can think clearly with you and act as your advocate in asking questions and writing down the doctors' responses. Why? Because most patients retain very little information when their circuits are overloaded by a serious diagnosis.

2. BE IN CHARGE

Create an equal partnership between you and your physicians (surgeon, oncologist, primary care doctor). Don't give up or just go along with medical decisions made by someone else. Ask your family and friends for support, but do not proceed with treatment just because they think it is the "right" thing to do.

3. KNOWLEDGE IS POWERFUL MEDICINE

Knowing the language of medicine will help you talk effectively with the medical specialists holding your future and make smart decisions about your treatment. You can become an expert in your illness—just as you may have learned about the financial world to invest in the stock market or the ins and outs of buying and selling on eBay. The availability of health information on the Internet can be your friend (or worst place to go). Stick with the Web sites operated by nationally known health groups and medical centers.

4. EXPLORE YOUR TREATMENT OPTIONS

Your doctor will lay out your options, but the buck stops with you. It's your decision which path you pursue. Ask the pros and cons of medication, surgery, chemotherapy, radiation, diet, and further sophisticated testing and clinical trials. Make sure you know the goal of treatment. Decide what you are "buying" with each option or combination of options. You *can* do nothing: one often-overlooked option is to accept *no* treatment or no *further* treatment.

5. ASK FOR A SECOND OPINION

When you're not satisfied with your diagnosis, treatment, or progress, you'll want to get a second opinion. Don't be shy. Recognize the importance of a second opinion. No single institution and no single physician or health care provider can have complete information about every condition. As professionals, they should not be offended if you want to seek a second opinion. This is a common practice in medicine today.

6. TAKE TIME TO TAKE YOUR BEST SHOT

Any serious diagnosis is devastating and paralyzing, so take time to think about your course of action before you rush to treatment.

With breast cancer, the signs and symptoms may have been present and undetectable for up to six years, not just since yesterday. Therefore, there usually is no real urgency to rush into treatment within a day or two of diagnosis. Keep in mind that many treatment options cannot be reversed. For example, removal of a breast is a major life-altering event.

Have some understanding of the natural history of your disease. Ask your doctor to explain the typical track record and progression. As with most situations in life, your first shot is the best. Gather all the information and opinions, and then make informed decisions to take your best shot.

7. SET UP YOUR SUPPORT SYSTEM AND KEEP EVERYONE THINKING POSITIVELY

Social connectedness is one of the biggest factors in explaining why some patients do better with serious illness than others. Well-controlled studies have shown that the support of family, friends and even pets lifts spirits mentally and boosts immune systems physically. Families need to be supportive of the patient's decisions—*no matter what those decisions are.*

8. DO NOT SECOND-GUESS YOUR HEALTH CARE DECISIONS

Don't look back. Plan ahead. Trust your instincts on your treatment, and maintain a comfort level with your care-providing team. If you don't think someone is acting in your best interest, get someone who is.

9. LIFE IS A FULL-TIME JOB—SET PRIORITIES

Time will take on new meaning. Make the most of it. Life when you're healthy is a full-time job. Be realistic when you're operating at less than 100 percent. Cut back. Slow down and smell the roses.

Nobody can go it alone, and now is the time to reach out and seek the help you need from friends and neighbors. Acknowledge the importance of a support system. A friend or confidante can be an anchor during some stormy times. Don't ignore the resources of your religious group, if you have one.

❧ *Think about . . .*
my treatment goal

❧ What is my diagnosis?

Know the type of breast cancer you have, its stage, grade and other characteristics. This information will help guide appropriate treatment options.

❧ Is my breast cancer curable or controllable or confinable?

Don't accept a response from your doctor of "we don't know." Doctors do know certain scenarios based on the experiences of similar groups of patients with the same type of disease. Each person's disease is different, but doctors can get in the ballpark.

❧ What are my chances of getting improvement from this treatment?

As you weigh your treatment decisions, you will want to increase the odds in your favor. If you aren't satisfied with the approach, response or positive outlook from your treatment team, seek a second opinion from another specialized medical center.

My Page

My Thoughts _____

_____

_____

_____

My Feelings _____

_____

_____

_____

My Facts _____

_____

_____

_____

My Support _____

_____

_____

_____

ξ

Leave 'em Laughing

Oh, my god, I have milk coming out of my breasts.
This is like having bacon come out of your elbow.
—CANDICE BERGEN AS MURPHY BROWN

A very dear friend of mine sent me a Christmas gift: stick-on nipples. They're made of silicone, but they didn't come with instructions or adhesives. My husband suggested, "Put a few drops of water on the back and maybe it will stick to your prosthesis."

I tried this, and it seemed to work. Why I thought my husband was an expert in the use of stick-on nipples remains a mystery to me.

I had to give a formal presentation at work, so I decided to take my new nipples for a test drive. I felt very risqué. I had on a silk shell, and I looked in the mirror and thought they were very subtle, but, oh yes, I could see them.

My presentation went well. I had slides, so I was doing a lot of pointing and arm waving. Afterward, I sat down next to a male colleague I hadn't seen for a year. It was hot, so I took off my jacket. I felt very pleased with myself in my sleeveless silk shell.

Coming around the table on a beautiful china plate were those Pepperidge Farm cookies. I reached over to take the plate from my colleague. Then I looked down at my little dessert plate, where I was supposed to place my cookie. There was already a cookie on it.

It was my left nipple.

So I'm sitting there, holding this heavy dessert plate, and the man looks at my plate and says, "Oh, I didn't see they had those thin wafer cookies. That's my favorite! Darn, it looks like you got the last one."

"It's my favorite too," I said. "I'm going to save it for later." In a flash, I grabbed the nipple and shoved it in my pocket. He looked at me like I was crazy.

My husband said later it was a good thing I grabbed it first or "that man would still be chewing."

♥ *Lillie Shockney, R.N., M.A.S.*

❡ *Think about* . . .
what to ask my doctor

- ❡ What's my treatment plan? What steps do I need to take and when?

- ❡ Tell me what you know about this cancer in general.

- ❡ Who can you recommend for an independent second opinion?

- ❡ Why is the treatment you are proposing right for me? What are my other options?

- ❡ If there are test results pending, how will I get the results? What steps do I need to take if the test is positive or negative?

- ❡ If surgery is involved, how many of these procedures have you performed?

- ❡ How long will it take me to recover from surgery, and what is the follow-up treatment?

- ❡ What clinical trials can I get into?

- ❡ Who is available to answer my questions, and how can I reach them?

꙳ Do you have support groups, psychologists and patient-to-patient programs?

꙳ What complementary therapies do you provide, such as music, art, yoga, meditation, spirituality?

꙳ Will my family be able to be involved in my treatments?

My Page

My Thoughts _____

_____

_____

_____

My Feelings _____

_____

_____

_____

My Facts _____

_____

_____

_____

My Support _____

_____

_____

_____

Barney

I n 1973 I was diagnosed with breast cancer. My mother had had a mastectomy in the '40s, and she had gotten along beautifully. I was a widow and the mother of two teenagers. My surgery and recovery went well, and I was able to return to work. I also volunteered as the Reach to Recovery person for our American Cancer Society.

When my first granddaughter, Heather, was about four years old, she was visiting my home overnight. I had to take a shower, so I had her stay in the bathroom with me.

When I was drying off, she noticed I had only one breast. She had lots of questions, and I tried to answer them to her satisfaction. Finally, she hung her head in deep thought and then asked, "Barney, if you have only one, why don't you wear it in the middle?"

♥ *Mary Ellen "Barney" LaFavers*

Talking About Breast Cancer . . .

"I have breast cancer." Some people will need to know (family, close friends, supervisor at work). Some people never need to know. But when you tell someone about your diagnosis, you may be surprised how much help and understanding comes pouring out.

With friends, family and coworkers:

- You'll find out who the true friends are—the ones who matter. They're the ones who just pitch in and do things for you, such as pick up the kids at school, bring over dinner and call just to listen.
- Pick one of those true friends—spouse, sister, best friend—to accompany you to doctor appointments and chemotherapy sessions. This is the person who becomes your eyes and ears, jots down what the doctor says, and helps you remember your questions and the doctor's answers.
- You don't have to act cheerful around others to make them feel more comfortable. Your closest friends will understand when you're too tired to talk.
- You may be amazed that the sister-in-law you never thought would be supportive becomes

your best friend. Or the complainer at work privately discloses to you that she too had breast cancer and offers to take you to her support group.

- Stay in touch with out-of-town family. Not knowing how you are is worrisome for them. Maybe start a family e-mail chat or designate someone to keep everyone else informed.
- Some people mean well but sure don't know the right things to say or do. Some friends will disappear. They may feel threatened, uncomfortable or fearful about cancer, and so be it.

If a friend, neighbor, coworker or family member truly wants to help you, give them a job—especially when you're exhausted and really need help. Women are accustomed to saying "no, thanks"; it's time to learn to say "yes, please."

With sexual partners:

Body changes and concerns about sex can affect the way you relate to your partner or how you feel about dating. As you struggle to accept changes yourself, you may also worry about how someone else will react to scars, a missing breast, sexual problems caused by medication, or just relate to someone who has "the big C."

- **Married?** Sexual problems can make feeling close especially difficult. Even for a couple that has been together a long time, staying connected can be a major challenge at first. It may be a comfort to learn that very few committed relationships end because of body changes. Divorce rates are about the same for people with and without a cancer history.

- **Single?** If you are single, you may wonder how and when to tell a new person in your life about your cancer and body changes. Fear of being rejected keeps some people from seeking the social life they would like to have. Others do not want to date and prefer to be alone but may face pressure from friends or family to "be more sociable."

Working Things Out at Work

A diagnosis of cancer and treatment should be handled at work just like any other illness. Take advantage of your sick leave, family and medical leave and short- and long-term disability. Work with your benefits coordinator to find out what the company health-insurance plan covers and even ask for a case manager to guide you over the months of treatment. Make your treatment decisions based on your own best judgment, not that of your insurance company or what is paid for and what is not.

Your coworkers will surely know about your diagnosis and may be some of your best advocates. But you will always want to be careful about disclosing your diagnosis to anyone else who has no need to know.

You and your doctor (not your boss) will decide when you can return to work—or whether you take any type of leave at all. Talk with your supervisor if you need accommodation such as flex time, work at home, ergonomic adjustments or special equipment to do your job.

If you find yourself pursuing a new job, you are not legally obligated to disclose your cancer history unless your past health has a direct impact on the job you seek. For example, if you have had a mastectomy and cannot lift any object weighing more than ten pounds with your right arm, you really don't want to be interviewing as a postal carrier.

❧

A Simple Door

*I've always believed that one woman's success
can only help another woman's success.*

—GLORIA VANDERBILT

A simple door separated two realities that ran parallel to one another. I stood on one side of the door with my recent diagnosis of breast cancer. I would have a mastectomy in four days followed by six months of chemotherapy.

On the other side of the door was my eight-year-old daughter, Alexandra, playing in her room. I knew that once I stepped over the threshold of her room, my reality would intersect with hers, and her life would change forever. I had postponed telling my daughter that I had cancer as long as I could, dreading having to say the words *cancer* and *mommy* in the same sentence.

I delicately pushed her door open just enough so I could see her. The little ringlets of hair fell softly around her face as she put a shiny black shoe on her doll. She looked up and saw me in the doorway. She smiled. I smiled back and moved to embrace her.

I could still remember what it felt like to live in innocence like hers, and longed to be back there. I sat down beside her, looked into her eyes and took her sweet, young hand in mine.

I said quietly, "I want to talk to you, honey. I have been diagnosed with breast cancer, and I'll be having surgery in four days to remove the cancer."

She looked completely perplexed. I could see that she was trying to understand the words I had just said. Then she was flooded with emotions. Her eyes filled with tears as the understanding of each word sank in. I held her and assured her I would be fine.

"Mommy, are you going to die?"

"No," I said. "The surgery and the chemotherapy will make me well."

Alexandra and I survived that day, and I went on to have my surgery and chemotherapy. My daughter was unwilling to speak about my cancer to her friends. Instead, she chose to keep her feelings to herself for several years.

When she reached adolescence, she began to talk more openly about her experience. I have come to understand that we will be talking about our relationship during that time, and my survivorship from cancer, for the rest of our lives. Each year brings a different, deeper conversation.

♥ *Lisa McPherson Robinson*

Share the Cancer Journey with Your Children

Children are often curious about cancer but are afraid to ask questions, so as a parent . . .

- Follow their lead. Honestly answer the questions they ask. It is important that you educate the child about everything that he or she wants to know.
- Find appropriate books to read with your child. It is important that the child has a clear understanding of what the disease is all about in terms he or she can understand. Your school librarian or child's teacher will have the best suggestions.

Major subjects to talk about with your child:

- **Fear.** Children fear losing a parent and the love, care and structure that a parent provides. Illness is frightening to children. Reassure your children that you love them no matter how bad you feel. Also reassure them that cancer does not mean you will die. Explain the different types of cancer.
- **Curiosity.** If your children are curious about what your surgery looks like, it is up to you to decide if you feel comfortable enough to

show them your scar. But remember, their imaginations may make it a lot worse than it really is.

- **Understanding.** Children need to know they have absolutely nothing to do with the cause of your sickness. The sickness you have is not contagious. Tell them age-appropriate facts about your treatment: how you will be treated, how you are feeling at the present time and how your treatment will change daily routines.

- **Relationships.** Tell your child that everyone's roles will change within the family, and the child will have to help more around the house.

- **Celebrate.** Give frequent updates on your condition. Celebrate the good days with a shopping trip, an ice cream cone, a walk in the park. Spend the at-home, in-bed days with a shared video movie or read a book together.

❧

Sisters at Last

An individual doesn't get cancer, a family does.
—Terry Tempest Williams

I told her she was adopted: such a cruel thing for a bossy eight-year-old to tell her innocent, little six-year-old sister. She cried. I loved it.

She wasn't adopted. We just had more photos in the family album of me, me, me, because growing up in the 1950s it was all about me. I hated my little sister.

I pushed her out of the tree swing. She plummeted awkwardly to the ground, landing on her arm. "Don't tell," I warned. She whimpered and sniveled and finally couldn't stand the pain any longer. She "told" and ended up with a very cool cast on her broken wrist.

As teenagers, I yanked her long hair so hard that I pulled out her pierced earring the painful, ugly way. I hogged the teen phone line. I laughed when she drove the car into a telephone pole. I reveled when she came home late to face grounding. And I raided her my-parents-aren't-home party and got her into big-time trouble.

As adults, we were openly civil but never close, so her divorce was a surprise, and I chose not to speak to her for a year over that. She remarried. They had a child.

"I had a breast lump removed; it's cancer," she announced. As grown women with kids and dogs and husbands who love us, we were finally on speaking terms, occasionally, even though I hadn't put her phone number on the speed dial. But now we talk a lot. Every single day.

She needs me, and I need her too. I'm her long-distance coach through medical decision making. We discussed the treatment options and researched the doctors together. We reviewed her ominous surgical and pathology report and cried over the lost breast. And we decided that because over half the women with this staging and diagnosis had a good outcome, she would surely be in that group. No question.

This time, if she falls out of the tree swing, I'm there to catch her. The big sister and the little sister. Sisters at last.

♥ *Sandra Goldberg*

People Helping People

Caregivers are often family members or close friends. Just like you, your caregivers need help and support. Here's how:

- **Build a team** so you don't have to depend on just one person.
- **Keep your caregivers informed.** Make a list of phone numbers of your medical care team, your pharmacy, friends, family, neighbors and spiritual leaders. Post this by the main phone. Make a list of all your medications, dosages and when you take them. Discuss your side effects and what you do about them. Make sure caregivers know if you have a living will, where your important papers are located and who has your power of attorney.
- **Take care of your caregivers.** Make sure they take time away from you to enjoy their own hobbies and run their errands. They need to take care of themselves to take care of you. Depression is common among caregivers. Encourage them to seek professional help if you see their spirits flagging.
- **Show that you care.** Let your caregivers know you value their help, support and love with a simple "thank you."

Tips for Caregivers

The trauma of cancer diagnosis and treatment will often send family members scrambling to rearrange roles, responsibilities and relationships. Navigating these new, evolving relationships takes communication, patience and support.

Readers of *CURE* magazine (Cancer Updates, Research & Education) offer this been-there-done-that advice for caregivers:

- **Always be optimistic.** Statistics have been proven wrong many times.
- **Be the patient's second set of ears.** This is critical when someone is newly diagnosed.
- **Be an advocate for your loved one.** Make sure his or her needs are met.
- **Keep your sense of humor.**
- **Know more than the patient** and provide nourishment to the patient in explaining what the doctors have said.
- **Be a little bit of everything:** psychologist, medical practitioner, spiritual guide, nurse and leader with a whole lot of unselfishness.
- **Rephrase the bad news** and intensify the good news.
- **Remember that when nothing can be said, touching says it all.**

- **Don't be afraid of emotions.**
- **Caregivers are a guidepost to the patient.** Patients can read your expressions.
- **Encourage friends and family to be a part of the care.** Don't be a warden; be a gatekeeper.
- **A caregiver must be a positive thinker and a curiosity seeker.** The caregiver many times will have to do work for both themselves and the patient.

And this patient-to-caregiver advice:

- **Lots of us will take as much attention** as you'll let us. Don't always fall for it.
- **You can still get mad at me** for not doing the dishes or forgetting to pay the mortgage.
- **Sometimes your positive energy** has to be enough for both of us.
- **Respect my self-esteem.** It's hard to accept the fact that I need to be cared for.
- **I don't want to feel fragile and helpless,** so respect my need for independence. Let me do as much for myself as possible.
- **Touch me.**
- **If you think I am overexerting myself,** check with my doctor before trying to keep me from living as normally as possible.
- **Take time for yourself.** Eat, sleep and exercise.

If you are tired and overburdened, you drag me down even farther.

- **Find the new person in me,** and let's learn to love and respect each other again.
- **Forgive me** if, in my fear of the unknown, I am difficult or unkind.
- **Remember to laugh and to cry with me.**
- **Be honest with me.**
- **Remember that we are human.** We have good days and bad days.
- **Most important, you can't do it all yourself.** Don't get lost in my cancer. Get support.

Breast Friends

One in seven women will get breast cancer in her lifetime. The other six will know her. And these are ways they can help her:

Just call to chat.

Hat shower: Give a shower for your friend. Have everyone bring a pretty or funny hat.

Take up a collection, and buy a day of house cleaning, window washing or carpet cleaning for your friend.

Cook a meal for her family on chemotherapy days.

Go to a matinee movie and/or to lunch.

Start a blog to keep far-away friends and family informed (it lessens the number of phone calls and e-mails to acknowledge). A blog is a running chat on a Web page.

Run some errands for her (grocery shopping, post office, bank deposits) or take her with you and double the fun.

Just call to chat.

Wash her car.

Help with yard work (and chat while working).

Arrange for a day of babysitting, so she can rest.

Go wig shopping—try on crazy colors (the crazier the better).

Invite her to a special lunch; bring out the fancy china and silver. Don't forget the linen napkins. What are you saving them for anyway? Celebrate your friendship and life.

Many restaurants have gourmet foods to go. Bring home her favorites, and enjoy them with her in comfy clothes.

Bring over an assortment of herbal teas. Looking for a better night's sleep? Try chamomile. Need an afternoon pick up? Try hibiscus and rose hips.

Just call to chat.

If your friend likes to cook, bring over some fresh herbs. Many supermarkets are stocking them these days.

Ice cream sundaes are always in style. Bring over a few toppings, and you have instant fun.

Create a fun "Do Not Disturb" sign for her to use if she needs some alone time. Great for the bathroom door to take that long relaxing bath or an afternoon nap. Don't forget a nice basket of bath products.

If you don't have time, pay a responsible teenager to do some mundane and tiring errands to take away some of the burden of chores (such as lawn mowing, dumping trash, raking leaves).

Breakfast in bed is always a hit. Don't forget the flowers to brighten up the tray.

Take your friend for a new look. It's more fun to do it together. If she's up to it, try on some new styles of clothes together. A bald head goes well with punk styles. Pick something you would never normally wear and have a good laugh. Don't forget the camera.

Get a few wild temporary tattoos and have fun putting them in daring places.

When you come to visit, suggest she take a relaxing aromatherapy bath while you watch the kids, do the dishes and laundry, or just field the phone calls.

Just call to chat.

Before she loses her hair, dye it a color she's always talked about, or get it cut short and sassy. Encourage her to be daring by trying out some new styles or looks. Remember, it's only going to last a week or so.

Try art therapy. Not creative enough? Bring over a couple of coloring books and crayons and help her feel like a kid again with coloring book therapy. It's a good time to talk and bring out the creativity even if she isn't an artist. Don't forget, it's okay to color outside of the lines.

If your friend is dealing with lymphedema, you could hire a massage therapist that is specially trained to help relieve the pressure and help her relax.

If you like to do crafts, bring over the supplies and share your craft with your friend.

Write "thank you" notes for her to acknowledge gifts.

If you have a sweet pet that likes people, share it with your friend. Pets have special healing power. (Check for allergies beforehand.)

One way to pamper your friend is to shampoo her hair (or massage her head with lotion if she has no hair).

If your friend lives a long distance from you, sign her up for "Fruit of the Month," or send Starbucks or other such gift cards, so she can enjoy a special treat, on you. Send flowers on the last day of chemo or radiation.

Oh, yeah . . . **just call to chat!**

♥ *Becky M. Olson and Sharon M. Henifin*

☧ *Think about . . .*
my caregiving team

- ❑ Spouse, significant other
- ❑ Mom
- ❑ Dad
- ❑ Sister
- ❑ Brother
- ❑ Daughter
- ❑ Son
- ❑ Mother-in-law
- ❑ Neighbor
- ❑ Teacher
- ❑ Family pet
- ❑ Friends
- ❑ Coworkers
- ❑ Church members
- ❑ Support-group members
- ❑ Religious or spiritual leader
- ❑ Fitness trainer
- ❑ Yoga teacher
- ❑ Massage therapist
- ❑ Hairdresser
- ❑ _____
- ❑ _____
- ❑ _____

✗ *Think about . . .*

who can I count on to . . .

✗ Carpool to my kids' events?

✗ Bring over a warm meal on days I don't feel like cooking?

✗ Drive me to treatment when I'm too tired to drive myself?

✗ Go for a shopping spree and leisurely lunch?

✗ Babysit? Run errands?

✗ Take care of chores and yardwork?

✗ Go with me to yoga class?

✗ Take a morning walk?

✗ Help me at work?

✗ Just be there to listen?

ƒ

Divine Inspiration

Your first emotion isn't
"Am I going to lose my breast?" It's
"Am I going to lose my life?"

—LINDA ELLERBEE, TV REPORTER

I really wanted my last radiation treatment to be special, for the radiation team as they were awesome, and for myself. Thirty-three days. Thirty-three treatments.

So I decided to bake biscotti—stayed up until 1:30 A.M., then got up early to package it, wrap it and write out cards. But something was missing. I wanted to be able to convey to the people at the hospital how much I appreciated them, their professionalism, their caring dedication, and how comforting it was to have them there during my treatments.

I also wanted my gift to be something memorable, something that would brighten their day and make me smile every time I thought about them. (The irreverent part of me just had to have the last word!)

All of a sudden, it came to me. It was inspired—it was brilliant—it was too stinking funny!

But I needed some help, and John had already left for work, so I called my neighbor and asked if she would come over.

When I arrived at the hospital, I changed and went into the treatment room. For thirty-three days, the technicians had carefully positioned me, lined me up with precision according to the tattoos and marks painted on my chest to make sure they treated the correct areas.

The technician came over to position me. He adjusted my drape, looked at me, looked again and burst out laughing. Another tech came in, looked, looked again and did the same thing.

I couldn't help it. It was too perfect. For some reason Bob Hope popped into my head that morning, and I knew it was divine inspiration. There on my chest, I had my neighbor write: *Thanks, for the mammaries.*

♥ *Mary Anne Breen*

Create a Mind-Body Focus

Use the power of your imagination. Visual imagery (mentally seeing yourself doing a task or being in a place) is like a dream. Athletes use it. Rock stars do it too. And regular practice has been shown to improve performance. If you use visual imagery, you can become more relaxed during a medical procedure, an X-ray, chemotherapy or before surgery.

How to: Close your eyes. Recollect a time you were extremely happy. Forget about everything else. Mentally enjoy the feeling of being in that event for at least ten minutes. Now open your eyes and feel the relaxation and recharging of your system.

Use the power of your voice. A centuries-old technique called chanting can generate mental and physical health benefits. Chanting is akin to singing, only you repeat the "song" over and over, either out loud or silently, alone or in a group. Chanting helps you withdraw your mental focus from worldly matters.

Chanting captures sound as vibration. Vibration creates power, just as high notes in songs have been known to shatter crystal. Chanting helps evoke the relaxation response, to break through your consciousness, which is essential to meditation. Through chanting, you take your mind to a healthier place and release helpful brain chemicals to elevate mood.

How to: Just chant the same word or phrase or song in the shower or even in the car, with or without a chanting music CD, as a way to insulate yourself from life's stresses or during a chemotherapy session.

ॐ

Heart Massage

*I call hope my "pilot light" because I now know
that, without it, we truly cease to exist.*

—VICKIE GIRARD

The first time I met Jeanne she was walking
down the path in front of my apartment, and I
was walking toward her. I noticed that she was
wearing a pink ribbon, and I was wearing mine too.
I stopped in front of her and said, "Wow, looks like
we have something in common."

She was taken aback and replied, "What do you
mean?"

"Well, you're wearing your pink ribbon and so
am I. Do you know someone who was diagnosed
with breast cancer?"

"Yes," she whispered. "Me." She walked away
quickly.

I'm a licensed massage therapist, and in my
work over the years I have seen many people in
pain. Recently I have been seeing a lot of women
with breast cancer.

A few days later I received a phone call from
Jeanne's husband. I had given him a massage the

year before when they visited my island home.

"I'd like to give my wife a massage as a gift and surprise her. She said she met you yesterday and had a good feeling about you."

When Jeanne walked into my massage room a few days later she seemed tense and angry. It was a warm, beautiful day, and her treatment had been a gift from her husband, so I was puzzled why she was upset.

"Are you feeling well?" I asked.

"My back hurts, and I'm a little nauseous."

And yet she was here and wanted to have her body massaged. I left the room, as I always do, to give her privacy for changing clothes and positioning herself on the massage table.

After I got her situated and the bed adjusted and my hands washed, I began by resting one hand at the base of her neck and the other on her lower back, allowing us both to become quiet.

In a calm voice, I suggested, "Let your eyes close and bring your attention to your breath." After several minutes I applied warmed lotion and gave light delicate stroking motions to her back and neck. I used long, slow movements to soothe her and encourage rest.

As I give a massage, I remind myself that there is nothing to "fix." I need only to "be present" with the person who is going through discomfort.

As soon as I turned her onto her back, her breathing became ragged, and she began to cry. I let her cry quietly for a while, and then asked, "Would you like me to incorporate mental imagery into the session?" She nodded.

"You can soften the discomfort you're feeling, and be open to it rather than push it away." That was all. No other words. Just "open" and "soften."

At the end of the treatment, as I was holding and stretching her neck, she began sobbing. I continued holding her without comment, allowing her a safe place to cry, to release, to heal.

While Jeanne was getting dressed she quietly but firmly said, "I would like to schedule at least one more treatment with you while I'm here in Maui. I recently had a double mastectomy. As part of my healing process I tried massage, but the therapist was clinical and cold, and the massage painful and traumatic. I was terrified to get another treatment—that's why I was so upset when I came here.

"I can't begin to tell you how much lighter in body and spirit I feel right now. And so connected. At the risk of crying all over again, I want to let you know how much you have helped me today to take that first huge step back toward allowing another human being to touch me . . . without fear or shame or remorse. Thank you."

It is an honor to be able to perform this type of healing work, and I was filled with a profound sense of grace and warmth. Light filled me. A completely transformed woman emerged from the massage session, and another transformed woman prepared her massage studio for the next client.

♥ *Pandora Kurth*

Think about . . .
coping with change

Women want to feel like women.
And you want to be feminine when you look
in the mirror . . . especially if you
are a single woman.

—SANDRA, BREAST CANCER SURVIVOR, 53

Are you concerned that others may notice hair loss, weight gain or loss of a breast?

Some body changes are short-term, and others will last forever. Either way, how you look may be a big concern after cancer treatment. Your feelings are natural, but one thing you have not lost is your sense of self.

Do you think others will act differently around you?

Changes in the way you look can also be hard for your loved ones—and this can be hard on you. Parents and grandparents often worry about how they look to a child or grandchild. They fear the changes in their body will scare the child or get in the way of their staying close.

⚹ Are you interested in ways to enhance your appearance during treatment?

If you find that your skin has changed color from radiation, ask your doctor or nurse about ways you can care for your skin and if the color will change over time. A new haircut, hair color, makeup or clothing may give you a lift. If you choose to wear a breast form (prosthesis), make sure it fits you well. Your health insurance plan may pay for it.

⚹ How are you really feeling?

Tell yourself that you are more than your cancer. Know that you have worth no matter how you look or what happens to you. Mourn your losses. They are real, and you have a right to feel the loss. Focus on the ways that coping with cancer has made you stronger, wiser and more realistic.

My Page

My Thoughts _____

_____

_____

_____

My Feelings _____

_____

_____

_____

My Facts _____

_____

_____

_____

My Support _____

_____

_____

_____

Hair Today, Gone Tomorrow

*When we are strong, we are always much greater
than the things that happen to us.*

—Thomas Merton

Heads up! One of the distressing downsides to many chemotherapies is that you'll lose your hair. The cruel joke is that you'll lose all your hair —EVERYWHERE—in places you don't want to lose hair, like your head, your eyebrows, your eyelashes and everywhere, and also in places you really wouldn't mind losing hair.

Most women are prepared to lose the hair on their heads in anticipation of months of really bad no-hair days, as if getting cancer, losing tissue or a breast or breasts isn't bad enough. But in trying to hold on to our sacred femininity we hate to lose our hair everywhere. We convince ourselves that our sexuality and sensuality are not located in our outward appearance but in our hearts and minds and spirits. It's just tough when you look in the mirror after surgery, chemo and radiation and some of our sacred parts are scarred, charred or missing.

In anticipation, you can cut your hair very short

and buy wigs (and have whatever hair color you always dreamed of). I had a girlfriend in charge of helping me pick out the best wig—then she cut and styled it to conform to my face. Caps and turbans work well too.

But there's just something too scary about looking in the mirror and dreading an alien staring back at you with no eyebrows. Two of my girlfriends shared my "eyebrow" concern. One went to the American Cancer Society's *Look Good, Feel Better* program with me so we could learn to use makeup to its fullest advantage during this stage of my treatment. The other girlfriend traced my eyebrows while I still had them and made me an eyebrow stencil.

If all else fails, go to the mall and throw yourself on the mercy of the ladies at the Estée Lauder cosmetic counter. They work miracles.

What I lost in hair, I made up for in earrings. My "wig director" made me some of the most gorgeous earrings you've ever seen. I decided that accessories restored a little of the flair I felt I was missing.

You'll spend time thinking about all the things you lose during breast cancer treatment, like hair. I did. But you'll also think about all you gain—prayers, family members and friends opening up about their love for you. Friends become wig directors and makeup consultants. Friends who never even cook for their own families bring over home-cooked meals and fill your freezer. One friend brought a pan of sand and seashells to a chemo session. I snuggled my feet into the warm sand and dreamed about being on the beach.

My hair has grown back. I have a different body and a different spirit now. I am better for all the love I have been given.

♥ *Kay Ryan, R.N., Ph.D.*

℟

The Long Journey

My husband and I went to Paducah, Kentucky, one Thanksgiving, to meet our son and his family who had come from Florida. They stayed in a motel with an indoor swimming pool.

After spending Thanksgiving Day with the family, the grandkids wanted to go swimming. My oldest grandson, Harrison, age six, asked, "Granny, can you come swim with me?"

"Yes," I said, and I got my swimsuit, prosthesis and a towel. Off we went.

Now, this swimsuit was not made for breast cancer women, so I just put my prosthesis in the cup of the suit. We walked down to the pool, jumped in, and swam to the steps. Harrison got out first and turned around to help me.

His eyes grew as big as saucers as his jaw dropped. He pointed at me and said, "Grandma, did you come from another planet?"

I looked down to where he was pointing and saw that my prosthesis had come out of the cup and slid down to my belly button.

"I've come a long way," I answered.

♥ *Bonnie Seibert*

The A-B-Cs
of Breast Forms

"The hardest thing about losing my breast was finding my stomach," said one woman recovering from breast cancer surgery. When you look down, past the soft arch of breast, irrespective of its size or shape—mercifully a little farther out than your stomach—you're not aware that you look pregnant. It's something about that middle-aged female stomach. Out of sight, out of mind.

Soon after breast surgery (and removal of one or possibly both breasts), a woman will consult with an expert trained in fitting a breast prosthesis. The idea is to make a woman look as much like herself as possible—so no one wonders which breast is missing. The secret is yours to keep.

Breast forms (or prostheses) are made of silicone—ironically, the same stuff used in breast augmentation. The form itself fits into a pocket built into a mastectomy bra and looks like and has the same weight as the existing breast. The forms come in various skin tones, including ebony for African American women.

Just because your insurance may cover the cost of two bras a year, don't think you *need* only two bras. With the selection of mastectomy underwear these days complete with matching panties, you'll want various colors, spaghetti straps, convertibles—every kind you wore before. Medically prescribed bras are sassier these days, with plenty of lace and underwire, so don't settle for something you're sure your old-maid grade-school teacher wore.

Did you know there's a medical reason to have a well-fitted breast form? If you don't replace the weight on one side or both, your body will change in response, just like if you had a tooth removed and other teeth shift to fill the gap.

Even a young woman needs to consider adding weight on the surgery side, because as she ages, subtle changes will occur. Her shoulder will begin to droop down and move forward, as if guarding the injured side. The changes are slight, but long term, and the imbalance may lead to back problems and osteoporotic curvature in the upper back.

If your missing breast was heavy, its loss will change your balance, so walking and being steady on your feet becomes an issue—especially for elderly women. The breast form evens out the weight.

For those backless-dress events (yes, you can do it!), breast forms that attach with special glue are ideal, but don't try these in your first year after surgery, before your incision completely heals.

If you think you can keep your old bathing suit, and just sew a pocket into it for the breast form, you may be all wet. Certain suits that highlight cleavage just aren't suitable for a breast form. But mastectomy bathing suits are stunningly fashionable, with a slightly different neckline.

If you've had both breasts removed, consider yourself lucky. Your biggest dilemma is settling on what size to be. Finally you, not nature, can decide to be an A, B, C or bigger. The best advice is to buy bigger breast forms as your waistline increases with middle age. You'll look proportionally thinner!

Shop at a boutique that caters to women's breast health needs. You will be assisted in privacy and comfort by a certified fitter. Breast cancer support groups can guide you to a shop near you.

Caution: Wear jewelry, pins and brooches on the side opposite the breast form or not at all. Imagine your surprise when the pin becomes unclasped and punctures your silicone form. No, it won't pop like a water balloon and cause a fashion emergency, but you might feel a slow, gummy leak down your favorite silk blouse.

ঁ

Angel Hugh

If you are going through hell, keep going.
—Sir Winston Churchill

"Try my feet," I groaned. "I've got some good veins there." The IV needle in my hand had stopped working, and an exhausted young doctor was unsuccessfully trying to insert a new one. She had been at it for half an hour. At midnight on a Friday, she was the only doctor on duty in the oncology ward of this National Health Service hospital in central London, and for me, she was the only game in town. I knew she'd been on duty for far too many hours, but I didn't really care. I had my own problems.

I growled, "I'll give you one more shot at it, then I'm done. I'll drink the damn blood, the antibiotics, the acyclovir, whatever you want. But after this one, I've had enough." I gritted my teeth, grabbed the cold iron bed frame and tried not to cry out. Vampira dug around, looking for a vein on my foot. She stabbed. She stabbed again.

"I can't do this," and she stood, hands shaking. "I've done twenty of these today, and I did them perfectly well. You've had so much chemo, and your veins just won't cooperate." She angrily pulled the curtain back and stomped out into the ward.

I had an infection in the central line they had surgically implanted in my chest, as well as an adverse reaction to my first high dose of chemotherapy. My white blood count had dropped, and a fever had gone so high that it gave me the shakes. I was at the nadir of my nadir. And all I wanted now was for it all to stop. All of it.

The last weeks had seen me in and out of the hospital in preparation for the high doses of chemotherapy I was soon to receive. Each visit meant a different bed, a different view of the same gray-green walls, and mostly different faces. Unlike American hospitals with their double or triple patient rooms, this was one large ward, with approximately twenty beds, separated only by the curtains you were allowed to draw 'round. It was a mixed-sex ward, but we had all lost our modesty along with our privacy. Personal dignity had somehow ceased to matter.

Most of my fellow patients were asleep, and I sat in my curtained cubicle, legs crossed, a red velvet hat on my bald head, listening to their snores and grunts. I dreaded the next chapter of my nightmare and had stopped trying to imagine just where the plot was headed.

Suddenly, the ward sister flung my curtain wide. "This is Hugh from the Intensive Care Unit." And she was gone.

"Nice hat," Hugh said with a grin, as he gently pulled the curtain shut. "Bet you're bald as a coot under there."

I tried to smile and failed.

"May I?" as he took a seat beside me on the bed. "What's the problem?" He looked me over, as though buying a used car. "I see a lot of places we can get a needle in." He counted the little Band-Aids plastered over all the failed attempts on my arm and hand.

"Thirteen," he exclaimed in wonder.

I shook my head. "You missed my feet."

He shook his head back at me. "And before every one, the doc said, 'This won't hurt a bit.' Right?" He laughed. "You ever hear the one about the guy who wanted to castrate his cat?"

I shook my head, slower this time. Was this guy going to tell me a joke? Didn't he have a life to save, a phone call to make, a nap to take?

Hugh continued. "He didn't have any money to go to the vet, so his best friend tells him, 'I'll do it for you. It's simple. You hold the cat. I get a couple of bricks, and I hold 'em one in each hand. Like this. When the cat's nice and calm, I do this.' And the best friend slams the two bricks together. The cat owner is appalled. 'Won't that hurt?' he whispered. 'Oh, no,' replied the best friend. 'Not as long as I remember to keep my thumbs up.'"

Hugh grinned even wider. And I laughed for the first time in days, as much at his enjoyment as at the joke.

In a low, conspiratorial voice, he went on, "So, the doc was right. It didn't hurt her a bit." I laughed again. "Now I'm going to numb this bit of your hand with a little cream, and we'll wait a minute for it to work. No need for any more pain than you have already, right?" We waited.

Hugh cocked his head. "They tell me you're having a hard time?" A pause, and he continued. "I had a Jeep accident in Africa a few years ago. My girlfriend and my friend were killed, and I was in the hospital for six months. It was a pretty dark time. It might have been something like what you're going through now." He was almost whispering. "You don't want to do this anymore, do you?"

I nodded, hesitantly. It was hard to admit in a world that admired fighters that I wanted to quit, to give up, to give in.

"I always compare it to *mal de mer*. You know, seasickness? When you're in the middle of a channel crossing to France, and the boat is heaving, and you're being sick over the side, all you want is for it to stop. You just want to die. But when you get to the other side, you can't believe you ever felt that way."

Hugh looked straight into my eyes. "You're going to get to the other side of this, and you won't believe you ever felt the way you've felt tonight."

I could feel tears drip down my cheeks. "Now, let's get this needle in. There. Done. Perfect." And it was.

He stood to go. "If you have any more trouble, have them page me, and if I'm in the hospital, I'll come." He stopped at the curtain and turned back. "I'm not a very good fortune teller, but I'm a heck of a good bookie. You know what I say? You're going to make it." With that, he was gone.

It's now seven years since I finished my high dose chemotherapy and the radiotherapy that followed. My health remains robust, and though others may say I am in remission, I consider myself cured. Out of my experience came my first play, *Gone to L.A.*, a black comedy about breast cancer, which will be made into a film later this year. In it, one of my favorite characters refers to "Angel Hugh from ICU," the guy who can "canulate your friggin' earlobe."

When *Gone to L.A.* opened at the Hampstead Theatre in London, I was pleased that a great number of the family and friends who helped me through my illness were among the audience. It made me laugh inside to know that Angel Hugh was one of them.

♥ *Lolly Susi*

More Than the Blues

After treatment, you may miss the support you received from your health care team. You may feel as if your safety net has been pulled away and that you get less attention now that treatment is over. Feelings like these are normal.

For most women with breast cancer, these feelings go away or lessen over time. But for one in four, these emotions can become severe.

When time does not heal the painful feelings, and your emotions get in the way of daily life, you may have a medical condition called clinical depression. Much more than the blues, depression is treatable with talk therapy, medications or a combination of both. Outcomes are excellent. For some breast cancer patients, cancer treatment may have contributed to this problem by changing the way the brain works.

Get help. You don't have to be a martyr, and there is nothing to be ashamed of. Talk to your doctor. If your doctor finds that you suffer from depression, he or she may treat it or refer you to other experts. Many breast cancer patients get help from therapists who are expert in both depression and cancer recovery.

These are the common signs of depression (and anxiety, a similar, treatable illness that often is the other side of the depression coin):

Emotional signs:

- A sense of being worried, anxious, blue or depressed that doesn't go away
- Emotional numbness
- Feeling overwhelmed, out of control, shaky
- A sense of guilt or worthlessness
- Helplessness or hopelessness
- Irritability and moodiness
- Difficulties concentrating, or feeling "scatter-brained"
- Crying a lot
- Focusing on worries or problems
- Not being able to get a thought out of your mind
- Not being able to stop yourself from doing things that seem silly
- Not being able to enjoy things any more, such as food, sex or socializing
- Finding yourself avoiding situations or things that you know are really harmless
- Suicidal thoughts or feeling that you are "losing it"

Physical symptoms:

- Unintended weight gain or loss not due to your cancer or treatment
- Insomnia or increased need for sleep
- Racing heart, dry mouth, increased perspiration, upset stomach, diarrhea

- Physically slowing down
- Fatigue that doesn't go away; headaches or other aches and pains not explained by your cancer treatment

Take Two Poodles and Call Me in the Morning

If you were stranded on a deserted island, would you want the company of your pet or another human? More than half of people surveyed by the American Animal Hospital Association chose their pets.

Your pet—whether you have a dog, cat, parakeet, iguana, even a horse—may be the answer to your feelings of frustration and worry, especially if the combination of breast cancer and depression are causing you to dwell on your problems. Pets keep you company, they keep you moving, they keep your mind off your aches and pains, and stroking them even releases brain chemicals that make you feel good. So never underestimate the power of your puppy!

My Page

My Thoughts _____

_____

_____

_____

My Feelings _____

_____

_____

_____

My Facts _____

_____

_____

_____

My Support _____

_____

_____

_____

ξ

A Cancer Therapist's Story

It's all right to cry, but not for too long.
I made it, and so can you.

—BETTY FORD

It was an unusual day at support group. For the first time in a long time, there were no newly diagnosed women present. In some coincidence of grace, all the women there that day were a year or more past treatment, none had recurred, and all were happy and in good health.

These were old friends. Women who had met when they didn't have hair or eyebrows. Women who had seen each other through the rough days of chemo sickness and radiation burns, shared the mounting panic of each follow-up visit, and rejoiced together with each "all clear" from an oncologist. These were the women who came to support group intermittently, whenever they could, not because they needed support but because they wanted to be there for the new women who had been forced into this sisterhood of breast cancer. Because their lives had picked up a normal pace again, many of them had not seen each other for months.

After the excited greetings and the normal catching up about health, lives, kids and jobs, a cozy, quiet reverie settled over the group. Each woman seemed to be soaking up the love and support and safety these friends offered, and the quiet was very comforting.

My job in these groups is to direct conversation and to observe. Today, I just listened.

Softly, Jeanne spoke up. "I've been thinking. If you could rewrite your life and redo the last few years, would you keep this experience? Would you do the cancer over again?"

The group was incredulous. They laughed.

"No way!"

"I wouldn't wish this on my worst enemy."

"You've got to be kidding!"

But Jeanne pushed on. I remembered when she wouldn't ever express an opinion. I was struck by her persistence, especially in light of the reactions she was getting.

"No, I don't mean would you choose to have cancer and be sick. I mean the whole experience. I've been thinking about how much this has changed me. I'm different. And I like the new me better. I was talking about this to my husband and I told him, if I could give back the cancer but I'd also have to give back all that I've learned, I think I would choose to keep it all. Of course, I NEVER want to do this again." She laughed.

Marge was nodding. "I think I know what you mean. My daughter was over visiting last week, and she said to me, 'Mom, don't take this wrong, but I like you better now.' That's a remark you have to follow up on. She never told me that before the cancer. Even though I always said she could talk to me anytime, she'd have to talk over the electric mixer or chase me around the house while I threw in laundry or made a bed. She said, 'Mom, now when I come over, you pour us a cup of coffee and sit down at the table and look at me. I feel like I really have you now.' I realized that she was right. I used to think I had to do it all; that it was all important. Now I believe that people are the most important. And I feel closer to my kids and friends now than I ever did before."

As the discussion went around the table, each woman added her own experiences of what she had gleaned from the cancer journey: a closer relationship with a husband, the courage to leave a boring job for something fun and interesting, a deep friendship that had developed during treatment. While many could never say they would choose to have cancer again, all could agree that they had changed and grown in ways they loved. They agreed that it is possible to go beyond just enduring the cancer experience; it is possible to transcend the trauma and weave the experience into the fabric of your life in a way that adds depth and character and beauty to the tapestry of your soul.

As the women left that day, I thanked God again for my job. Every day I get to see the very best of the human spirit that rises up in the very worst of times. I thought of my own mother, who had breast cancer in the days before Betty Ford, before support groups, before the word *cancer* could be said aloud. I wondered how different her cancer experience would have been if she had had the opportunity to share it with women like these.

I was so grateful to all of the women who had the courage to rip the stigma of shame and secrecy away from breast cancer; to the women who are willing to tell their stories, so other women will not have to suffer alone; and to the wonderful women who are able to create beauty and strength from shards of shattered health.

♥ *Stephanie Koraleski, Ph.D.*

✗ Think about . . .
is a support group right for me?

- ✗ Do you like being part of a group?

- ✗ Do you like to talk about your feelings with others?

- ✗ Do you want to hear stories about other people and their cancer?

- ✗ Are you looking for helpful hints, or do you want to share your advice?

- ✗ Would such a group make you feel better?

The number one reason people join a support group is to be with other people who have "been there"—not because they do not receive support from friends and family.

How to Find a Support Group

Support groups come in all shapes and sizes: breast cancer only, all types of cancer, women only, families, certain racial and ethnic groups, led by breast cancer patients or led by medical professionals.

Other groups focus on family issues surrounding cancer, relationships, financial worries, and supporting a family member with breast cancer.

Start with your doctor and cancer nurses. Your cancer treatment center will have a community listing. Hospital community relations coordinators and social workers are often the leaders or set up meeting rooms. Your local newspaper may have general listings.

Check in with your local chapter of the American Cancer Society and other cancer-related organizations. And if you visit a women's health care boutique, they will have listings of groups, events (such as the Susan G. Komen Race for the Cure), and all kinds of fund-raising activities.

Meet in cyberspace. Not only do support groups meet in person, they also meet in online chat rooms. These Internet support groups can be a big help if you live in a rural or remote area or prefer the privacy of an electronic identity. With Internet groups, you can seek support at any time of the day or night.

While these groups can provide valuable emotional support, they may not always offer correct medical information. Be careful about any cancer information you get from the Internet.

Use caution when comparing cancer stories and treatments. What's right for someone else may not be right for you. Check with your doctor before making any treatment, dietary or activity changes based on what you read or hear in any group.

My Page

My Thoughts _____

_____

_____

_____

My Feelings _____

_____

_____

_____

My Facts _____

_____

_____

_____

My Support _____

_____

_____

_____

✗

You're Gonna Eat That?

*Strength is the capacity to break a
chocolate bar into four pieces with your bare
hands—and then eat just one of the pieces.*

—JUDITH VIORST, AUTHOR

In case you're wondering where to hook up with a bunch of breast cancer survivors, you may find them in the natural foods section of the supermarket, scouring labels for traces of soy.

Like beauty queens who are expected to uphold the standards of the pageant as they travel the world on their goodwill tours, breast cancer survivors are often expected to be paragons of healthy eating. I flinched before bacon and smoked meats for a long time after my diagnosis, muttering such things as "unclean!" and pulling my shawl tighter around my face like a vampire at the first streaks of dawn.

In fact, one of the first things I did while under the influence of the steroids I got along with chemo was to throw out everything in my kitchen.

"I don't know what poisoned me, but I'm getting rid of it!" I said in my steroidally induced 3 A.M. frenzy. Never mind that breast cancer can strike even if you're mainlining phytoestrogens; I had to blame *something*, and closest at hand were frying pans encrusted with what I believed to be carcinogenic evidence. I admit now it is much more likely that I simply wanted to justify a spending spree at Williams-Sonoma.

Breast cancer survivors are attracted to the idea of impeccable eating habits mainly because we feel betrayed by our bodies. But there's pressure on us from other sources as well, thanks to that famous study of Japanese women who, when they moved to Hawaii and changed their diet to a fast-food American one, developed a higher incidence of breast cancer. We still don't know precisely what in an American diet produced this effect (although I'd put my money on "supersizing"), and we don't know for sure precisely what about their former diets may have protected the women. Although everyone assumes it's soy, I'm hopeful it's the tempura.

The initial rush to culinary perfection can be very heady. For six months, I was a vegan, which is a vegetarian who doesn't eat . . . well, who doesn't eat anything: no meat, fish, eggs, dairy, just a lot of tofu pies disguised as chicken, and visits to restaurants where everything on the menu is in quotes, like "cheeseburger" or "BLT."

Being a vegan was not onerous for the time I was

devoted to it. What was more annoying than a life without cheese was when I went back to normal eating, and other people looked at me like, "You had breast cancer and you're gonna eat *that?*" Just as politicians are expected to be monogamous and movie stars are expected to roll out of bed perfectly beautiful, breast cancer survivors are expected to set a culinary example. And the people criticizing us are often the ones with steak juice running down their chins.

I think it's because they've displaced their own fears on us about getting cancer. Everyone wants a talisman to ward off disease, and just as it was easier to blame my cancer on my kitchen equipment or eating habits, people are comforted to think we can control our fates through healthy eating.

Unfortunately, vegetarians get breast cancer too, so this theory is not without its holes. But human nature persists. The next time you order something doused in butter and someone gives you the evil eye, tell them to go sit on a rice cake and mind their own business. Even beauty queens only have to serve for a year. Then they get to live the way they want, with or without a tiara on their heads like a halo.

♥ *Jami Bernard*

Essential Truths About
Healthy Eating

In the process of killing cancer cells through chemotherapy and radiation, healthy cells that divide rapidly are also damaged, especially those in the mouth (and hair, but that's another story). This process causes side effects that might affect your ability to eat.

Forget fad diets, restricted calories, or any diet, for that matter. It's essential to eat well and as nutritiously as possible. Now's the time to go for the gusto with foods higher in calories and loaded with protein. Even if you're concerned about your cholesterol level, a hot fudge sundae won't sabotage your eating habits. In other words, if it sounds tasty, go for it. The idea is to build up your strength to help you withstand the rigors of treatment.

- Drink or eat more milk, cream, cheese and cooked eggs.
- Use sauces and gravies, and include more butter, margarine or oil.
- Try new foods. Some things you may never have liked before may taste good to you during treatment.
- Stock the pantry and freezer with favorite foods so that you won't need to shop as often.

Include foods you know you can eat even when you are sick.

- Keep foods handy that need little or no preparation, for example, pudding, peanut butter, tuna fish, cheese and eggs.
- Do some cooking in advance and freeze meal-sized portions.
- Your appetite may be better in the morning. Eat your main meal then, and try liquid meal replacements (such as Ensure or Boost) later if you don't feel like eating.
- Eat what appeals to you, without thought to being well balanced. Try to include plenty of protein.
- Drink fluids (fruit punch, sports drinks, soft drinks and vegetable broth are some new choices), especially if you don't feel like eating.

℥ Think about . . .
side effects

Do you have:

℥ Loss of appetite?

Try frequent, smaller meals, snacks and smoothies, and simply eat when you feel hungry. A small glass of wine or beer may stimulate your appetite. Carry a canned meal replacement with you in case hunger strikes.

℥ Weight loss?

When you eat, pack in as many calories as you can (use whole milk, real full-fat ice cream and add dried milk as protein powder to anything you eat, such as eggs, soups and sauces). Think peanut butter.

℥ Weight gain?

Certain breast cancer medications and hormone therapies may cause weight gain. If the gain is from water retention, your doctor may prescribe a diuretic (water pill). If the gain is from what you're eating, well, back to low-calorie nutritious eating. And exercise.

☧ Sore mouth or throat, tender gums?

Chewing and swallowing may be difficult, so substitute soft foods such as mashed potatoes, milkshakes, malts, smoothies, yogurt, custard, pudding, scrambled eggs, oatmeal and anything you can puree in your food processor. Avoid hot foods. Suck on ice chips, and talk with your doctor and dentist about special toothpaste and soothing mouth rinses.

☧ Dry mouth?

Chemo and radiation tend to reduce the flow of saliva. Carry a water bottle and sip all day. Tart foods and beverages such as lemonade may stimulate more saliva. Popsicles are soothing. Moisten dry foods before you chew them. Use a soft toothbrush, and rinse with warm water.

☧ Changed sense of taste or smell?

Foods, especially meat or other high-protein foods, can take on a bitter or metallic taste. Other foods may have less taste. Boost flavor with sweet marinades or seasonings such as basil, oregano, rosemary, orange or lemon. Try using bacon, ham or onion to add flavor to vegetables.

Nausea?

Nausea often strikes a few days after chemotherapy. Your doctor can prescribe excellent drugs to combat nausea given at the beginning of a chemo session and then taken when needed. Choose foods easy on your stomach, such as oatmeal, angel food cake, skinless chicken, canned peaches, soft drinks and ice chips.

Diarrhea?

Eat plenty of foods and liquids that contain sodium (chicken broth) and potassium (bananas, mashed potatoes), two important minerals that help your body work properly. These minerals are often lost during diarrhea. Sports drinks such as Gatorade contain both sodium and potassium and have easily absorbable forms of carbohydrates.

Too tired to eat?

Feeling tired during cancer treatment can be related to a number of causes: not eating, inactivity, low blood counts, depression, poor sleep and side effects of medicine. Plan on your energy level being half of what it normally is. Build naps into your day, and get a good night's rest. Eat when you are hungry.

What's Your Alternative?

Are you thinking about taking vitamins, minerals or other dietary supplements, such as herbs, not prescribed by your doctor?

The National Cancer Institute strongly urges breast cancer patients to depend on traditional, healthy foods. Too much of some vitamins or minerals can be just as dangerous as too little. Large doses of some vitamins may even stop your cancer treatment from working the way it should. To avoid problems, don't take these products on your own. Follow your doctor's guidance.

My Page

My Thoughts _____

_____

_____

_____

My Feelings _____

_____

_____

_____

My Facts _____

_____

_____

_____

My Support _____

_____

_____

_____

✄

Diagnosis: Canceritis

When you think about it, what other choice is
there but to hope? We have two options, medically
and emotionally: Give up or fight like hell.

—LANCE ARMSTRONG, ATHLETE, CANCER SURVIVOR

I t was just a little bump. A little red mosquito-bite-looking bump on my stomach, and I discovered it while I was taking a shower.

I have skin tags, moles, beauty marks, age spots and other "skin decorations" too insignificant to have names, but I'd never had one on my stomach. I didn't think about it again.

Until the next day. Again in the shower, I noticed the little red bump, but then forgot about it once I turned off the water.

On day three, when the bump hadn't gone away, I started getting nervous. I found myself surreptitiously lifting my shirt throughout the next couple of days to check it, and every time it was still there I became more alarmed.

I tried to talk myself down and stay calm. But each time my fingers felt that slightly raised spot, my heart skipped a beat.

I lived in a steadily increasing state of panic for seven long days and then did what any woman who had just finished breast cancer treatment would do: I got to my doctor's office as fast as I could!

When I had been diagnosed with breast cancer, I immediately thought I was going to die. And pretty soon. But as the days and weeks passed, I realized I just might be one of the lucky ones who made it and so began to relax a little.

By that time, I was fully engaged in my treatment plan and doing everything possible to be well again. I tried to cover all the bases: combining conventional medicine's chemo, surgery and radiation with not-so-conventional treatment like meditation, visualization and dance movement therapy. I became an expert in my kind of breast cancer and drove my oncologist crazy with questions about bizarre therapies I'd found on dubious Web sites.

I felt like I had a handle on this cancer thing, like I had some control.

Then, after nine months of total immersion in medical appointments, procedures and theories, focused only on my healing, I finished treatment.

Wow! I was ecstatic and relieved that I had survived all the poking and prodding and probing and plotting. Now, I thought, my life can get back to normal: no more treatments or doctor appointments or tests.

The euphoria of finishing treatment lasted a week. Then it hit me that I was no longer doing anything to keep the cancer away. I felt like a tight-rope walker performing without a net.

I became obsessed with checking for signs that *it* was back. Breast self-exams were not enough: I performed total body exams. Cysts I'd had for decades became suspect. Moles that had been part of my physical landscape from birth were examined daily for changes. Showers became agonizing events as I scrutinized every inch of my body for evidence that *it* had taken over again. I had a full-blown, hard-core case of "canceritis."

Yes, canceritis—the most common and least treatable long-term side effect of breast cancer.

I first encountered canceritis shortly after I was diagnosed. I was on the phone with my mother, a forty-five-year survivor, and she was telling me how funny her surgeon was all those years ago when she'd gone through her breast cancer experience. She laughed as she recalled one visit when, after listing for him all her aches and pains that proved the cancer had returned, he asked her where she'd received her medical degree. I remember rolling my eyes and thinking how incredibly paranoid she was.

So, a few months later, here I was doing the same thing over a little red bump! And I wasn't the only one. I'd met many women who had survived breast cancer, and every one of them had canceritis. Some called their doctors daily with "symptoms," some just thought about calling, but all of them were preternaturally aware of every nuance of their bodies. And their "symptoms" had begun shortly after their treatment had ended.

Hair grows back, nausea goes away—the body heals. But the mind gnaws on that cancer thing like a dog gnaws on a bone: compulsively for a time and then burying it, digging it up, burying it, digging— again and again. There are many medications and therapies to heal the body's wounds, but only one treatment for the mind. The magic bullet for alleviating the symptoms of canceritis is time. And the more time that passes, the less canceritis you have.

Forty-five years later, when my mother gets a cough, her first thought is not, "Oh, my God, I have lung cancer." After all the years and colds and coughs and various ailments, the possibility that the cancer's come back is pretty far down the list of "what it could be." Forty-five years of time has cured my mother of canceritis.

However, it had been only forty-five days for me when I found that little red bump on my stomach. The doctor said it was nothing. I asked how she knew it was nothing. She said it didn't look like cancer, didn't feel like cancer, wasn't in a logical place for cancer to be. I repeated my question. She explained that just because I've had cancer doesn't mean I'm not a candidate for other illnesses and conditions (hardly fair, if you ask me). And I said that sounded reasonable, but how did she know it was nothing.

Just to get rid of me she sent me to the dermatologist—who told me it was nothing. I asked how she knew it was nothing. She said it didn't look like cancer, didn't feel like cancer, wasn't in a logical place for cancer to be. I repeated my question. Just to get rid of me, I think, she removed that little red bump, did a biopsy of it and proved that it was indeed nothing.

I felt a lot better without that little red bump on my stomach (of course, now there's a little red scar instead), but I realized how foolish I'd been. It's understandable that I would immediately suspect cancer, and it was responsible of me to consult a doctor, but I did go a little overboard, insisting on a second opinion and a biopsy. That canceritis definitely had me going.

So, I've decided to take a lesson from my mother and think twice before diagnosing myself with cancer every time I have a little ache—or a little red bump. And I've decided to stop the anatomical examinations in the shower every day. Why go looking for trouble? Why live the rest of my life worrying about every little something that pops up?

And I plan on making those changes just as soon as I get back from the doctor. You see, I've got this pain in my finger and . . .

♥ *Lori Misicka*

The Continuing Challenge:
Fearing Cancer's Return

How do you cope with fear of cancer returning? Here are some ideas that have helped others deal with fear and feel more hopeful:

DO I KNOW WHAT TO LOOK FOR?

Learning about your cancer, understanding what you can do for your health now and finding out about the services available to you can give you a greater sense of control. Some studies even suggest that people who are well informed about their illness and treatment are more likely to follow their treatment plans and recover from cancer more quickly than those who are not.

WHERE CAN I EXPRESS MY FEELINGS OF FEAR, ANGER OR SADNESS?

Being open and dealing with their emotions helps many people feel less worried. Women have found that when they express strong feelings like anger or sadness, they are more able to let go of these feelings.

Some sort out their feelings by talking to friends or family, other cancer patients, or a counselor. Of course, if you prefer not to discuss your cancer with others, you should feel free not to. You can still sort out your feelings by thinking about them or writing them down (journaling).

Thinking and talking about your feelings can be hard. Some people just want to move on. While it is important not to let cancer "rule your life," it may be hard to avoid. If you find cancer is taking over your life, it may be helpful to find a way to express your feelings. Art and music are expressive ways.

HOW CAN I WORK TOWARD HAVING A POSITIVE ATTITUDE?

Sometimes this means looking for what is good even in a bad time or trying to be hopeful instead of thinking the worst. Use your energy to focus on wellness and what you can do now to stay as healthy as possible.

Don't blame yourself for your cancer. Some people believe that they got cancer because of something they did or did not do. Not true. Cancer can happen to anyone.

You don't need to be upbeat all the time. Many women say they want to have the freedom to give in to their feelings sometimes. As one woman said, "When it gets really bad, I just tell my family I'm having a bad cancer day. I cancel all my appointments. I go upstairs and crawl into bed."

- **Find ways to help yourself relax.** The exercises in this book, including chanting and visual imagery, plus listening to healing CDs

have proved to help others and may help you
relax when you feel worried.

- **Be as active as you can.** Getting out of the
  house and doing something worthwhile can
  help you focus on other things besides cancer
  and the worries it brings.

WHAT SHOULD I DO WHEN I FEEL OUT OF CONTROL?

Control what you can. Some women say that
putting their lives in order makes them feel less
fearful. Being involved in your health care, keeping
your appointments and making changes in your
lifestyle are among the things you can control. Even
setting a daily schedule can give you more power.
While no one can control every thought, some say
they've resolved not to dwell on the fearful ones.

WHAT'S THE BEST THING FOR ME TO DO RIGHT NOW?

Your best defense is early detection: breast cancer
may return in the same breast, the other breast, or
set up a beachhead in another part of your body,
such as your lungs, liver or brain. A recurrence is
not a new cancer. It's considered the same as your
original breast cancer, even though it may show up
elsewhere. For some reason, a small number of
cancer cells may have survived the initial treatment

(surgery or chemotherapy or radiation or a combination) and took time to grow into tumors large enough to be detected.

You may find signs of them after weeks, months or many years. That's why it's important to have regular cancer checkups on a schedule you set up with your doctor.

My Page

My Thoughts _____

_____

_____

_____

My Feelings _____

_____

_____

_____

My Facts _____

_____

_____

_____

My Support _____

_____

_____

_____

The Alchemist

I am riding alone in a ferris wheel seat, locked in, with no choice but to go with the flow. Drawn up, riding backward, not knowing where I am going, but trusting that someone, somewhere, is guiding my journey.

The answer was there when I had the consultation. I saw the look on their faces. I heard their words, but I did not believe them. Smiling, I said, "Sure, wait until I get to the top of the ferris wheel . . ."

This didn't make sense to me. I was 27, married for a year and a half and no history of breast cancer in my family. The big question kept reeling through my mind: Why?

I was afraid to move, afraid to breathe, afraid to touch the beautiful place on my body that now had a wound. I knew the reality of what had happened. I just didn't want it to come alive. Does anybody know who I am and how I feel? I have just lost a part of my body. Who will love me now? Will I die?

All I could see from my hospital window was a small piece of cloudy sky, a reflection of glare and old red brick buildings. I am still alive even though I am encased like a mummy who has lost her femininity in layers of gauze and heavy surgical tape. I closed my eyes to sink into the lovely comfort of the anesthetic cloud that held me in its arms. I would be all right! It was February 1973.

"Yes, I am very hungry today. Aren't you?" I smiled at my friend as we walked down the hall toward our offices with big containers filled with salads from the hospital cafeteria. I was feeling great this day in May 1982 having just completed my annual medical exams with flying colors. Proud I had gotten past the five-year mark to beat the statistics and then the seven-year mark where I could actually say in a whisper, "I had breast cancer."

Now I had the goal to make 10 years and beyond. I was going to be the finest role model, showing every woman she could survive breast cancer.

"Monica," said the chief of surgery at Johns Hopkins, where I was working in cytopathology. "I need to see you and your husband in my office. When would be the best time to make an appointment?"

My inner knowing said, "Uh oh, something does not feel good. I don't like this."

My mind, body, brain, and mouth were all detached from one another. I felt myself talking but couldn't remember what I said. I felt myself halfway smile out of politeness and began to feel a warm ripple of courage from my British-Scots-Irish-German ancestry toughen up inside, readying myself for a mysterious battle. Yes, of course a time and date. I would call his office right away.

My God, what was going to happen to me now? I have a life to live, children to birth, a husband to love, dreams to realize. No, no, not again. I had bought another ticket on the ferris wheel.

Waking up from this surgery was a snap. I sailed through having another part of my body artistically removed, but the prognosis was even better. Surely this time I was home free.

I knew inside that this would be the end of this chapter of my life. I was going to be all right. Without a doubt I had a knowing about this. Now my body felt balanced; I felt healthy; now I was saved from the jaws of defeat; now I could begin my next new life.

My two breast cancer events changed my view of life in many ways. The evolution from viewing these experiences as living a horror story to receiving a gift was not done overnight but involved a process of commitment, perseverance, trust, and love. There would be many facets of these events that would bring me closer to my life's purpose and therefore my soul's evolution.

These experiences taught me that receiving gracefully was as significant as giving. Receiving allows others the honor of giving of themselves to you. I learned more about giving compassion to myself on a higher level, for example, by living and enjoying each moment fully through all of my senses and feeling proud and fulfilled for every effort I made to take care of myself during the most life-threatening circumstances.

How could my loving God do these horrific things to me? I had wailed, cried, sobbed and gulped for air, unable to find a decent logical answer. In exhaustion and filled with fear, I almost gave up.

But God wanted me to expand my options and horizons beyond what my human mind had planned. He wanted to develop a stronger partnership with more clarity so that I could receive the master plan for my growth toward wholeness and freedom.

I am not a victim anymore. I am the victor of my life.

♥ *Monica D. Traystman, Ph.D.*

It's Back, Now What?

Nothing is more devastating—not even the first time you heard the words, "You have cancer."

Your cancer is back. The shock is back. The fears are back—of telling your family and friends, of more treatment, and possibly of death. The anger is there too. You may feel that after all you've been through, it should have been enough. And the unanswered question is, "Will the treatment work this time?"

Even though you may feel some of the same things you felt when you were first diagnosed, now there is a difference. You've been through this before. You've faced cancer and its treatment and the changes that came to your life. You know that medical care and emotional support are available to you. Facing cancer again is difficult, but it's a challenge you can handle.

Breast cancer may return in the same breast, the other breast, or set up a beachhead in another part of your body, such as your lungs, liver or brain. A recurrence is not a new cancer. It's considered the same as your original breast cancer, even though it may show up elsewhere. For some reason, a small number of cancer cells survived the initial treatment (surgery or chemotherapy or radiation or a combination), and took time to grow into tumors large enough to be detected.

You may find signs of them after weeks, months, or many years. That's why it's important to have regular cancer check-ups on a schedule you set up with your doctor.

Starting cancer treatment again can place demands on your spirit as well as your body. Your attitudes and actions really can make a difference. Remember that you've coped with this situation before. Keeping your treatment goals in mind may help you keep your spirits up during therapy.

As you go through treatment, you're bound to feel better about yourself on some days than on others. When a bad day comes along, try to remember that there have been good days, and there will be more. Feeling low today doesn't mean you'll feel that way tomorrow or that you're giving up. At these times, try distracting yourself with a book, a hobby, or plans for a new garden. Many people say it helps to have something to look forward to—even simple things like a drive, a visit from a friend, or a telephone call.

What to Do

✗ Ask questions. Of your doctor, of support groups, of information forums at hospitals. Of the American Cancer Society. Of trusted online information sources. Learn about clinical trials.

✗ Tend to the legal aspects. Having a will and signing a living will designating a medical power of attorney and access to your bank account are things best settled in the beginning, rather than later, when you may be too ill.

✗ Plan for the best; prepare for the worst. The transition from active treatment to supportive care isn't easy. It takes time for a patient to accept the fact of impending mortality.

Adapted with permission from *CURE* magazine *(www.curetoday.com)*.

My Page

My Thoughts _____

_____

_____

_____

My Feelings _____

_____

_____

_____

My Facts _____

_____

_____

_____

My Support _____

_____

_____

_____

Close the Door When You Leave

I never asked you to visit . . . at least I don't
    believe I did
Maybe . . . I don't know
It's so confusing

At any rate, you're a rude guest
You take my energy, rob my sleep, and with a stick
You swirl and distort my dreams

All right; You are here—for now
But understand
There are two places that are forever off limits

You may not tread on my spirit
You may not occupy my soul

I have heard of your visits to others
I know the damage you leave in your path
The wanton disregard for innocence, value, and
    what some would call fairness

Also, I hear that laughter confuses you; that good
    foods make you feel bad, and

That nothing causes you more distress than an
     autumn sunset, the forever blue of a summer sky,
Or the unconditional radiance of a child's smile

Listen and understand
You might pilfer my closets, empty all the drawers,
     and trash my house
But there are two places forever off limits

You may not tread on my spirit
You may not occupy my soul

Do not mistake my nausea, weakness, and pain as
     signs of your victory
They are simply small dents in the armor I wear
     to fight you
Instead, look deeply into my eyes

They will once again remind you that there are
     two places forever off limits

You must not . . .
May not . . .
Will not tread on my spirit

You must not . . .
May not . . .
Will not occupy my soul

♥ *Michael Hayes Samuelson*
(male breast cancer survivor)

§

Abreast in a Boat

*Women agonize over cancer; we take as a personal
threat the lump in every friend's breast.*

—MARTHA WEINMAN LEAR, AUTHOR

Normal morning practice for the Pink Phoenix dragon boat crew was a half-hour paddle up Portland, Oregon's Willamette River and then back downstream. On March 25, 2000, the elite paddlers were engaged in time trials on the river, while our crew of newbies in the sleek, ornate shell of another boat was simply trying to get the timing right.

The Pink Phoenix club was formed in 1997 to demonstrate the high quality of life for women surviving breast cancer. We all have a story to tell about diagnosis, treatment and survival. But we don't dwell on our cancer stories. We come together in our own unofficial support group with paddles on water in competitions and for fun. Although dragon boating may soon be an Olympic sport, for us the camaraderie and sisterhood are enough. We are survivors, and we are already winners.

But no one realized that chilly March morning

what it truly meant to be survivors, all pulling together in the same boat.

Instead of heading upriver, our new crew was so uncoordinated, we seemed to be paddling in circles. We never made it up the usual river route. We were instead swinging around the nearby Ross Island Bridge to head back to dock when several of us saw a flicker of red fall from the bridge to the water.

"What was that?"

"My God, it's a man!"

Instantly, the caller said, "Paddles up, ladies. Let's go get him." Miraculously coordinated, synchronized, we efficiently closed the gap to the figure bobbing in the water.

Four of us were trained health care professionals, so we yelled back and forth about how to handle a rescue.

"Stay put. Don't reach out."

The nurse in me was screaming caution at the same time I took off my pink life vest and passed it forward.

"Don't stand up."

If we stand up or try to haul someone into our tipsy, fragile shell of a boat, we'll all end up in the water.

"Poke him with a paddle."

"Is he alive?"

By the time we sculled to our victim, threw him

a rope and pulled him alongside our gunwale, he was delirious and hypothermic, mumbling, "I'm sorry. I'm so sorry." He had jumped from the 500-foot bridge into bone-chilling 50-degree water.

Dave, a thirty-something meth addict who felt life was no longer worth living, found himself lifted up, literally hearing voices of what he thought were angels. Some angels we were: a motley crew of women ranging in age from thirty to sixty who had suffered surgery, chemo and radiation, whose lives had been turned upside down by breast cancer, and who had lost breasts, hair and husbands. We all survived. And some unseen hand had guided our boat to be positioned for a rescue. He was a lucky man indeed.

I stay in touch with him. When we paddle on the Willamette in festivals, we sometimes see him along the shore cheering our pink boat. He's still trying to plan a career after serving in the military, a disappointing divorce and several failed jobs that led him to jump to his death—only to find rebirth in our boat. Dave still struggles to keep his head above water and find happiness in his life. But he knows we're there for him, holding a rope, if only he will grab the other end.

♥ *Fern Carness, R.N., M.P.H.*

What Your Doctor Won't Tell You About Breast Cancer's Mysterious Complication

Doctors don't talk about it, but a condition called lymphedema may develop anytime you have a lumpectomy or mastectomy, have lymph nodes removed, or undergo radiation treatment for breast cancer.

The reason many doctors don't discuss lymphedema is because no one really knows what might trigger the condition after breast cancer surgery or other treatment. Lymphedema may develop right after surgery—or years after treatment.

What exactly is lymphedema? It's a fluid build-up in tissue, usually in the arm next to the breast that was removed or surgically treated. If lymph glands were removed, lymphatic fluid may not have open channels to freely flow throughout your body (*edema* means swelling). Especially if you have an injury or cut prone to infection, the body's defenses may trigger more lymph than your channels can handle, and swelling is excessive. Fluid then collects in tissues of the affected arm and causes swelling. Sometimes the increase in the size of the arm and fingers can be dramatic.

Physical therapists perform specialized massage

to keep fluid moving (and you can learn to do this yourself), but you must be vigilant about protecting your at-risk arm. With proper care and vigilance, you can avoid lymphedema or keep it under control. Here are some smart suggestions:

- Be gentle, dry thoroughly after a bath or shower, and don't wear tight rings or bracelets.
- Wear gloves when gardening to avoid cuts or scratches. Take care when cooking to avoid burns. Be vigilant about cat scratches or dog bites.
- Protect yourself from sunburn with long sleeves and sunscreen.
- Avoid saunas and hot tubs with their extremes of temperature (or drape your arm out of the hot tub). That includes hot baths and dishwater too.
- Wear a medical alert bracelet or necklace that says **LYMPHEDEMA ALERT: No blood pressure, no needles into this arm**. Choose an alternate spot for IVs or blood draws. Your thigh is an alternative place for blood pressure to be taken.
- Let someone else lift heavy items for you, including luggage (or use bags with rollers). Carry a heavy purse on the other shoulder.

- Pamper yourself with a manicure, but don't trim your cuticles. An electric razor may be the best way to shave under your arms to avoid nicks.
- When flying, wear a pressure sleeve (available at breast specialty shops and medical supply or pharmacy locations) well fitted to your arm. Changes in altitude and cabin pressure may trigger lymphedema in a woman who has never had a hint of it before. Drink plenty of water when flying too.
- For more information, contact the National Lymphedema Network (NLN) at *www.lymph net.org*.
- Always call your doctor if you notice any swelling, rashes, itching, pain or fever.

Row, Row, Row Your Own Boat

Avoid vigorous exercise. You might bring on lymphedema. That was the thinking among medical professionals. But studies are showing that vigorous exercise—even as intense as rowing—was not only doing no harm, it was giving women who had breast cancer surgery the aerobic and bone-building benefits they needed. Because chemotherapy brings on premature menopause, women who undergo this treatment are at increased risk for heart disease and osteoporosis (bone thinning). Competitive sports restore bone density and are good for your heart—and your soul.

Sometimes You Just Get Lucky

*The goal is to live a full, productive life . . .
the important thing is that the days that
you have had you will have lived.*

—GILDA RADNER

Why me? I have asked that question more times than I care to count over the past twenty-two years, and the only answer that makes any sense is "sometimes you just get lucky."

I am a four-time breast cancer survivor and have lived with cancer for most of my adult life. I know little else—I have no sense of how my life might have been without cancer. Everyone's life has a rhythm: get the kids up and off to school, hurry to work, rush to the supermarket after work to buy food for the next day's breakfast, check homework, get kids to bed on time, then collapse into bed to recharge for another day.

My life rhythm is almost identical, but it includes another element that those spared from breast cancer will never know. Regular visits to the oncologist, scans, X-rays, ultrasounds, biopsies, surgeries, breast reconstruction, implants, chemotherapy, radiation, tamoxifen, reading and researching, blood tests and more. It's a carefully choreographed movement that develops its own rhythm. Get the kids up, rush to work, visit the oncologist, get blood work done, pick up the toaster waffles, check homework, read the latest findings on a new and promising drug or vaccine, then bedtime for all.

That is my life. Most wouldn't trade theirs for mine, whatever the price, yet I wouldn't trade places with them either. I don't always catch the green lights or choose the quickest line at the supermarket. But how could I not feel lucky?

I'm fifty-one years old and still here! Since my first diagnosis of breast cancer many years ago at the age of twenty-nine, I've had the privilege of waking to 8,030 mornings. I've celebrated twenty-two birthdays. I carried, delivered, nurtured and raised two beautiful children, now in their teens, who show great promise for a bright future. I played a mean game of tennis for years. I jumped for joy at the publication of my first children's book. I've learned to sail. I have a house with a view of the water. All this, while living with breast cancer. How could anyone think my life has not been lucky?

Friends and family have told me often that they could never go through what I've been through. This statement is a curious one. I want to ask, "Would the alternative be better?"

Somehow, when faced with adversity, strength pays you a visit. It invites itself in and begins its transformation on your inner being. Emotions, resolve, the will to win, all of which have been at a constant simmer, begin to boil and erupt with a determination to beat this challenging opponent.

Does everyone win? Sadly, no. But you must try with a vengeance to ensure you'll be here to do whatever it is you're destined to accomplish. My belief in that thought kept me going through each biopsy or chemotherapy treatment. I knew my journey had miles to go, and I couldn't give up without my best effort.

People often ask me, "If you could relive your life, would you change anything or wish to be cancer free?"

My answer is always no. Everything that has happened to me, including having had cancer four times, has led me to this exact place in my life. There is a reason why my life evolved the way it did. Someday I hope to learn that reason.

Has cancer been easy? Not always. Did it change my focus? Absolutely! Has it forced me to stop and pay attention to the important things in my life? Without question. And I wouldn't change a thing. I like a good challenge, and I'll take luck wherever I can get it.

♥ *Arlette Braman*

Resources

On line health information is not a substitute for your doctor's advice. But it can sure make you a smarter patient when you see your doctor. You can know the medical terms, the tests, the procedures and treatment options and be able to discuss these issues and your concerns with your doctor—by starting your conversation on a higher level.

The National Cancer Institute of Canada is a one-stop source for patient education (*www.ncic.cancer.ca* and 416-961-7223)

Health Canada provides articles, research and statistics on breast cancer. (*www.hc-sc.gc.ca/english/diseases/cancer.html* and *www.phlc-aspc.gc.ca/ccdpc-cpcmc/bc-cds/index_e.html*)

Alternative Medicine College of Canada links you to relevant information at *www.alternativemedicine.com*

Canadian Cancer Society, *www.cancer.ca,* 1-800-268-8874

Breast Cancer Care & Research Fund, *www.breastlink.org*

Breast Cancer Research Foundation,
www.bcrfcure.org

Breast Cancer Survivors' Club (Mothers
Supporting Daughters with Breast Cancer),
www.mothersdaughters.org

TheBreastCareSite.com,
www.thebreastcaresite.com

Breast Friends, *www.breastfriends.com*,
888-386-8048

Facing Our Risk of Cancer Empowered (FORCE),
www.facingourrisk.org, 866-824-RISK (high genetic
risk, BRCA mutation)

Living Beyond Breast Cancer, *www.lbbc.org*

National Breast Cancer Coalition,
www.natlbcc.org, 202-296-7477

National Breast Cancer Foundation,
www.nationalbreastcancer.org

National Lymphedema Network,
www.lymphnet.org, 800-541-3259

Sisters Network, *www.sistersnetworkinc.org*,
713-781-0255 (serving African American women)

Susan G. Komen Breast Cancer Foundation,
www.komen.org, 800-I'M-AWARE, supporting
Race for the Cure

WHO Foundation (Women Helping Others),
www.whofoundation.org,
800-WHO-4-ONE

Y-ME National Breast Cancer Organization,
www.y-me.org, 800-221-2141 (interpreters in 150
languages)

Canadian Breast Cancer Foundation,
www.cbcf.org

Breast Cancer Society of Canada, *www.bcsc.ca*,
1-800-567-8767

Canadian Breast Cancer Network, *www.cbcn.ca*

Breast Cancer Action, *www.bcaott.ca*,
613-736-5921

Canadian Cancer Advocacy Network,
www.neutropenia.ca

Women's Cancer Network, *www.wcn.org*,
604-877-6187

Who Is Jack Canfield,
Cocreator of *Chicken Soup for the Soul*®?

Jack Canfield is one of America's leading experts in the development of human potential and personal effectiveness. He is both a dynamic, entertaining speaker and a highly sought-after trainer. Jack has a wonderful ability to inform and inspire audiences toward increased levels of self-esteem and peak performance. He has authored or coauthored numerous books, including *Dare to Win, The Aladdin Factor, 100 Ways to Build Self-Concept in the Classroom, Heart at Work* and *The Power of Focus.* His latest book is *The Success Principles.*

www.jackcanfield.com

Who Is Mark Victor Hansen,
Cocreator of *Chicken Soup for the Soul*®?

In the area of human potential, no one is more respected than **Mark Victor Hansen**. For more than thirty years, Mark has focused solely on helping people from all walks of life reshape their personal vision of what's possible. His powerful messages of possibility, opportunity and action have created powerful change in thousands of organizations and millions of individuals worldwide. He is a prolific writer of bestselling books such as *The One Minute Millionaire, The Power of Focus, The Aladdin Factor* and *Dare to Win.*

www.markvictorhansen.com

Who Is Edward T. Creagan, M.D.?

Edward T. Creagan, M.D., is an oncologist at the Mayo Clinic and a professor at the Mayo Clinic College of Medicine. He holds two endowed chairs as the American Cancer Society Professor of Clinical Oncology and Rouse Professor of Humanism in Medicine. He is the author of *How Not to Be My Patient: A Physician's Secrets for Staying Healthy and Surviving Any Diagnosis* (published by HCI Books, 2003) and *Mayo Clinic on Healthy Aging.* An engaging and endearing presenter, he speaks to audiences throughout the country on health promotion, patient empowerment, career burnout and cancer. Contact Dr. Creagan through his Web site: *www.HowNotToBeMyPatient.com.*

Who Is Mary Olsen Kelly?

Mary Olsen Kelly holds a master of fine arts degree in theater and spent the first twenty years of her adult life working in the entertainment industry as a writer, producer and director of television (notably P.M. magazine), video and theater. She was one of the founding advisors and members of the Inside Edge, one of the premier inspirational speaking organizations on the West Coast. She edited an encyclopedic anthology on New Thought Literature called *Fireside Treasury of Light* and cowrote *Finding Each Other: How to Attract Your Ideal Life Mate* with her husband, Don Kelly. Her most recent book is *Path of the Pearl: Discover Your Treasures Within*. The observations in *Path of the Pearl* stem from Kelly's experiences as co-owner of a chain of fine jewelry stores specializing in pearls and in overcoming such life obstacles as in relationships, financial difficulty and cancer.

Who Is Sandra J. Wendel (writer)?

Sandra J. Wendel, a consumer-health writer and editor, collaborated with Dr. Creagan on *How Not to Be My Patient*. She develops health content for *eMedicineHealth.com* and her own company's online health content at *www.Health-eHeadlines.com*. She is editor of the Wise Women Speak book series, *www.wise-woman-health.com*.

More Chicken Soup

Many of the stories in this book were submitted by readers just like you. If you would like more information on submitting a story, visit our Web site at *www.chickensoup.com*. If you do not have Web access, we can also be reached at:

Chicken Soup for the Soul
P.O. Box 30880, Santa Barbara, CA 93130
Fax: 805-563-2945

Sources

Lawrence LeShan, Ph.D., is a psychotherapist who has worked with cancer patients for over forty years. His research has led people with cancer to find new, effective ways to fight for their lives. Psychological change, along with medical treatment, mobilizes a compromised immune system for healing. Dr. LeShan and his colleague **Ruth Bolletino, Ph.D.**, can be reached through their Web site, *www.cancerasaturningpoint.org.*

Alan Pritz is a practitioner and teacher of Eastern disciplines who is based in Minneapolis. He is founder and president of Inner Resource Enhancement and Center for Inner Awakening (*www.CSpiritAwake.com*). He is the author of *Pocket Guide to Meditation* and has produced a CD of devotional chants, *Joy of the Soul: Cosmic Chants.*

Contributors

Jami Bernard is an author, humorist and award-winning film critic for the *New York Daily News*. She is the author of four film books and *Breast Cancer: There & Back* (Warner Books), about battling the disease (successfully!) in 1996. Her sixth book, due in bookstores January 2006, is a humorous memoir on how she lost 100 pounds by embracing a healthy lifestyle. Jami resides in New York with Sensei, the parrot, and cats, Tsuko and Buzz. The parrot can bark and the cats chirp. You can visit her Web site at *www.jamibernard.com*.

Arlette Braman is a freelance writer with many articles to her credit and the author of six nonfiction children's books. When not working, she indulges in her passion—sailing on the Chesapeake Bay. Arlette lives in both Pennsylvania and Maryland and enjoys quality time with family and friends. She is a four-time breast cancer survivor. Contact Arlette via e-mail at *arlnb@mac.com* or at her Web site, *www.arlettebraman.com*.

Mary Anne Breen—former Miss Colorado USA, model, cruise line sales manager, mortgage loan officer—finally found unlimited opportunity as an independent business owner with her husband, John, and son, Connor. She credits God's grace, her Christian community, family, friends, business mentors—all who helped her breeze through eight chemo and thirty-three radiation treatments. If she ever thought her breasts would one day get her in a book, she wasn't thinking cancer! She now cherishes all her titles: Wife, Mother, Survivor. Contact her at *heart2hand@covad.net*.

Fern Carness, R.N., M.P.H., C.M.F., a women's health advocate, is co-owner of Just Like a Woman, a retail experience in Portland, Oregon, that blends specialty lingerie needs with health education and survivor support services. Fern is a gold-medal paddler who represented the United States Senior Women at the 4th World Dragon Boat Championships and was awarded the Medal of Valor from the City of Portland along with her dragon boat crew for the rescue described in this story. She is publisher of the Wise Women Speak series (*www.wise-woman-health.com*).

Stephanie Koraleski, Ph.D., is a licensed psychologist in the Behavioral Health department at Omaha's Methodist Health System. She is a certified hypnotherapist, Reiki master, and student of healing touch and EMDR. Her current practice includes people diagnosed with cancer and other life-changing illness. She is a frequent presenter on mental health and mind-body topics and contributing author to the Wise Women Speak series (*www.wise-woman-health.com*).

Pandora Kurth lives in Maui, Hawaii. She has been a licensed massage therapist for over fourteen years, dedicated to her work in the healing arts. Although licensed in many different techniques, she uses the Hawaiian Lomi Lomi technique, where her massage table becomes sanctuary and Divinity touches humanity. Before moving to Hawaii, Pandora lived in Southern California where her parents, married over fifty-four years, and six siblings still reside. Pandora loves to travel, garden, read, write, snorkel and spend time with her loved ones.

Mary Ellen "Barney" LaFavers, a retired nurse who lives in Somerset, Kentucky, was diagnosed with breast cancer over thirty years ago. She's a mother, grandmother and now great-grandmother who likes to crochet and read. Her nickname "Barney" was an affectionate derivation from her maiden name during nurse's training and has stuck ever since.

Lori Misicka is a professional speaker who helps people of all kinds bounce back from adversity of all kinds. Her down-to-earth techniques were developed during twenty years of managing customers and staff in the broadcast industry and put to the test when she was diagnosed with breast cancer. Contact her at *lori@howtofeelgoodwhenyoufeelbad.com* or 916-402-0583.

Becky M. Olson and **Sharon M. Henifin** are cofounders of Breast Friends, a cancer outreach group in Portland, Oregon. Becky is a professional speaker and author of *The Hat That Saved My Life*. She lives in Beaverton, Oregon, with her husband, Bill, and their dog, Gretchen. Sharon is a computer and sales trainer and travels extensively in her work. She lives in Tigard, Oregon, with her husband, Vern, daughter Chelsea and her two cats, Onyx and Jake. Contact them through *www.breastfriends.com*.

Michele V. Price has lived and worked in Oregon since 1979. She is a seventeen-year breast cancer survivor who during her healing process learned that literature, writing and creative imagination can transform people and teach them to live well and to die well. She has had poems published in *Verseweavers* and *Manzanita Quarterly*.

Vicki Rackner, M.D., F.A.C.S., a member of the National Speakers Association, is a board-certified surgeon and clinical instructor at the University of Washington School of Medicine. After diagnosing and treating surgical patients for ten years, she left the operating room and formed her own company, Medical Bridges (*www.medicalbridges.com*), to inspire and empower people to make consistent choices that lead in the direction of health and wellness. Dr. Rackner is the medical editor of the nation's most widely read employee health newsletter, *The HOPE Health Letter*.

Lisa McPherson Robinson lives with her daughter in Bethesda, Maryland. She has been a psychotherapist in private practice for twenty-two years. Lisa believes she learned how to live by almost losing her life. Each new day spent with her daughter is a precious gift. She can be reached at *www.lisamrobinson.net*.

Kay Ryan, R.N., Ph.D., is the proud mother of Jamie, Kara and Kevin and grandmother of Emily. She lives in the house she grew up in, in Omaha, Nebraska. Kay is the vice president for institutional effectiveness at Nebraska Methodist College. Kay presents internationally on the topic of holistic health and plays the bodhran (Irish drum) in O'Carolan's Consort, an Irish band. She's a contributing author to the Wise Women Speak series.

Michael Hayes Samuelson is a nationally recognized author, social commentator and motivational speaker. The Lance Armstrong Foundation, The Patient Advocate Foundation and St. Jude Children's Research Hospital are among the scores of organizations where Michael has delivered his inspirational message. He also serves as a guest host for the American Cancer Society's Cancer Survivor Network and, at the request of former President George H.W. Bush and Mrs. Bush, is a member of C-Change. Michael is himself a breast cancer survivor. He is author of *Voices from the Edge, Moments. . . . Not Years,* and *What Would Mickey Say? Coaching Men to Health & Happiness.* His books can be ordered from *www.CancerCarePackage.com.*

Bonnie Seibert is an eight-year survivor of the disease that took her mother and sister. She participated in a clinical trial to help other women, including her sisters. She is an active member of the breast cancer survivor group in her hometown near Lexington, Kentucky, and likes to quilt, sew and sing in her church group.

Lillie Shockney, R.N., M.A.S., an award-winning, nationally recognized expert and inspirational speaker on breast cancer, is a breast cancer survivor and author of the *Breast Cancer Survivor's Club: A Nurse's Experience* and *Joining the Club: The Reality of Breast Cancer.* She is administrative director of the Johns Hopkins Breast Center. She co-founded a nonprofit organization called Mothers Supporting Daughters with Breast Cancer (*www.mothersdaughters.org*).

Lolly Susi, an American, lives in London. She graduated from Tufts University and trained at the Central School of Speech and Drama. Her acting credits include London's West End, BBC-TV and radio. Her films include *Dirty Rotten Scoundrels, Proof* and *The Jacket.* Lolly also directs professionally. As a writer, her first play was produced by the prestigious Hampstead Theatre in London. She has two new plays, both set in Maine, and is presently writing a book about the Central School of Speech and Drama, which is due out in 2006.

Monica Traystman, Ph.D., a molecular geneticist by training at Johns Hopkins, is president of Healthy Spirit, Inc., and Inner Light Coaching in La Jolla, California (*www.iamahealthyspirit.com*). Her company develops and presents seminars, workshops and retreats to promote and maintain a balanced mind, body and spirit. She is a life coach, primordial sound meditation instructor, trained at The Chopra Center, a certified Reiki master, a Self-Esteem and Peak Performance seminar facilitator, and hatha yoga instructor.

NOTES

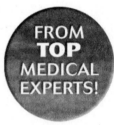